Equality, Diversity, and Inclusion in Sports Medicine

Editors

CONSTANCE R. CHU
ERICA TAYLOR
JOEL BOYD

CLINICS IN SPORTS MEDICINE

www.sportsmed.theclinics.com

Consulting Editor
MARK D. MILLER

April 2024 • Volume 43 • Number 2

ELSEVIER

1600 John F. Kennedy Boulevard • Suite 1800 • Philadelphia, Pennsylvania, 19103-2899

http://www.theclinics.com

CLINICS IN SPORTS MEDICINE Volume 43, Number 2
April 2024 ISSN 0278-5919, ISBN-13: 978-0-443-18197-9

Editor: Megan Ashdown
Developmental Editor: Malvika Shah

Clinics in Sports Medicine (ISSN 0278-5919) is published quarterly by Elsevier Inc., 360 Park Avenue South, New York, NY 10010-1710. Months of issue are January, April, July, and October. Business and Editorial Offices: 1600 John F. Kennedy Blvd., Ste. 1800, Philadelphia, PA 19103-2899. Customer Service Office: 3251 Riverport Lane, Maryland Heights, MO 63043. Periodicals postage paid at New York, NY and additional mailing offices. Subscription prices are $390.00 per year (US individuals), $100.00 per year (US students), $430.00 per year (Canadian individuals), $100.00 (Canadian students), $504.00 per year (foreign individuals), and $235.00 per year (foreign students). For institutional access pricing please contact Customer Service via the contact information below. Foreign air speed delivery is included in all *Clinics* subscription prices. All prices are subject to change without notice. **POSTMASTER:** Send address changes to *Clinics in Sports Medicine*, Elsevier Health Sciences Division, Subscription Customer Service, 3251 Riverport Lane, Maryland Heights, MO 63043. Customer Service (orders, claims, online, change of address): Elsevier Health Sciences Division, Subscription Customer Service, 3251 Riverport Lane, Maryland Heights, MO 63043. **Tel: 1-800-654-2452 (U.S. and Canada); 314-447-8871 (outside U.S. and Canada). Fax: 314-447-8029. E-mail: journalscustomerservice-usa@elsevier.com (for print support)**; **journalsonlinesupport-usa@elsevier.com (for online support)**.

Reprints. For copies of 100 or more of articles in this publication, please contact the Commercial Reprints Department, Elsevier Inc., 360 Park Avenue South, New York, NY 10010-1710. Tel.: 212-633-3874; Fax: 212-633-3820; E-mail: reprints@elsevier.com.

Clinics in Sports Medicine is covered in *MEDLINE/PubMed (Index Medicus) Current Contents/Clinical Medicine, Excerpta Medica,* and *ISI/Biomed.*

Contributors

CONSULTING EDITOR

MARK D. MILLER, MD, PE, Colonel USAF (Ret)
S. Ward Casscells Professor Emeritus, Head, Division of Sports Medicine, Department of Orthopaedic Surgery, University of Virginia, Charlottesville, Virginia; Team Physician, James Madison University, Founder, Miller Review Course, Harrisonburg, Virginia

EDITORS

CONSTANCE R. CHU, MD
Professor and Vice Chair Research, Department of Orthopedic Surgery, Stanford University, Redwood City, California; Department of Orthopedic Surgery, Stanford University, Stanford, California

ERICA TAYLOR, MD, MBA
Vice Chair of Equity, Diversity, and Inclusion, Duke Department of Orthopaedics, Duke Health Integrated Practice Chief Medical Officer of Diversity, Equity, and Inclusion, Orthopaedic Hand Surgeon, Duke University School of Medicine, Duke Fuqua School of Business, Executive in Residence, Faculty, Founder and CEO, Orthopaedic Diversity Leadership Consortium, Wake Forest, North Carolina

JOEL BOYD, MD
Orthopedic Surgeon, TRIA Orthopedic Center, Bloomington, Minnesota

AUTHORS

LAUREL A. BARRAS, MD
Department of Orthopaedic Surgery, University of Virginia, Charlottesville, Virginia

CONSTANCE R. CHU, MD
Professor and Vice Chair Research, Department of Orthopedic Surgery, Stanford University, Redwood City, California; Department of Orthopedic Surgery, Stanford University, Stanford, California

DAVID R. DIDUCH, MD
Professor, Department of Orthopaedic Surgery, University of Virginia, Charlottesville, Virginia

STEVEN FRICK, MD
Professor Department of Orthopedic Surgery, Stanford University, Stanford, California

CHASE GAUTHIER, MD
Research Fellow Department of Orthopedic Surgery, Prisma Health, Columbia, South Carolina

JEFFREY GUY, MD
Professor, Department of Orthopedic Surgery, Prisma Health, Columbia, South Carolina

RAM HADDAS, PhD
Assistant Professor Department of Orthopedics and Rehabilitation, Center for Musculoskeletal Research, University of Rochester Medical Center, Rochester, New York

SOMMER HAMMOUD, MD
Associate Professor, Department of Orthopaedics Rothman Orthopaedic Institute, Philadelphia, Pennsylvania

MARY L. IRELAND, MD
Associate Professor-Clinical Faculty, University of Kentucky, Lexington, Kentucky

EMMA E. JOHNSON, MD
Rothman Orthopaedic Institute, Philadelphia, Pennsylvania

PRAMOD KAMALAPATHY, MD
Department of Orthopaedic Surgery, University of Virginia, Charlottesville, Virginia

STEPHANIE KHA, MD
Resident, Department of Orthopedic Surgery, Stanford University, Stanford, California

JASON L. KOH, MD, MBA, FAAOS, FAOA
Mark R. Neaman Family Chair of Orthopaedic Surgery, Director, Orthopaedic and Spine Institute, NorthShore University HealthSystem, Illinois; Clinical Professor, The University of Chicago Pritzker School of Medicine, Chicago, Illinois

JUSTIN KUNG, MD
Resident, Department of Orthopedic Surgery, Prisma Health, Columbia, South Carolina

AMY LADD, MD
Elsbach-Richards Professor of Surgery and Professor, by Courtesy, of Medicine (Immunology & Rheumatology) and of Surgery (Plastic and Reconstructive Surgery), Department of Orthopedic Surgery, Stanford University, Stanford, California

MICHAEL D. MALONEY, MD
Dean's Professor of Orthopaedics and Physical Performance, Chief of Sports Medicine, Founder and Director of CHAMPP, Department of Orthopedics and Rehabilitation, Center for Musculoskeletal Research, University of Rochester Medical Center, Rochester, New York

WILLIAM J. MALONEY, MD
Boswell Chair of Orthopaedics Department of Orthopedic Surgery, Stanford University, Stanford, California

TIMOTHY A. McADAMS, MD
Clinical Professor Department of Orthopedic Surgery, Stanford University, Stanford, California

KELLIE K. MIDDLETON, MD, MPH
Northside Hospital Orthopaedic Institute, Lawrenceville, Georgia; Board Certified Orthopaedic Surgeon, Shoulder and Sports Medicine Fellowship Trained, Northside Hospital, Atlanta, Georgia

SHAUN NELMS, EdD
Department of Orthopedics and Rehabilitation, Center for Musculoskeletal Research, University of Rochester Medical Center, Rochester, New York

ALANA O'MARA, BS
Medical Student Department of Orthopedic Surgery, Stanford University, Stanford, California

GABRIELLA E. ODE, MD
Orthopaedic surgeon Department of Orthopaedics, Hospital for Special Surgery, New York, New York

KATHERINE RIZZONE, MD
Assistant Professor Department of Orthopedics and Rehabilitation, Center for Musculoskeletal Research, University of Rochester Medical Center, Rochester, New York

EDWARD M. SCHWARZ, PhD
Professor, Department of Orthopedics and Rehabilitation, Center for Musculoskeletal Research, University of Rochester Medical Center, Rochester, New York

KEVIN SHEA, MD
Orthopaedic surgeon Department of Orthopedic Surgery, Stanford University, Stanford, California

ERICA TAYLOR, MD, MBA
Vice Chair of Equity, Diversity, and Inclusion, Duke Department of Orthopaedics, Duke Health Integrated Practice Chief Medical Officer of Diversity, Equity, and Inclusion, Orthopaedic Hand Surgeon, Duke University School of Medicine, Duke Fuqua School of Business, Executive in Residence, Faculty, Founder and CEO, Orthopaedic Diversity Leadership Consortium, Wake Forest, North Carolina

PEDRO J. TORT SAADÉ, MD
Surgery Department, Doctors' Center Hospital San Juan, Doctors' Center Hospital Orlando Health-Dorado, Orthopedic Surgeon, San Juan, Puerto Rico; Associate Professor, Universidad Central del Caribe School of Medicine, Bayamon, Puerto Rico, President of the Tort Orthopaedic Institute, San Juan, Puerto Rico

ALEX TURNER, BS, BA
MD Candidate, University of Texas Southwestern Medical School, Dallas, Texas

MAIKE VAN NIEKERK, PhD, MD Student
Department of Orthopedic Surgery, Stanford University, Stanford, California

AUGUSTUS A. WHITE III, MD, PhD
Ellen and Melvin Gordon Distinguished Professor Emeritus of Medical Education and Professor Emeritus of Orthopedic Surgery at Harvard Medical School, Boston, Massachusetts

JOANNE ZHOU, MD
Resident Department of Orthopedic Surgery, Stanford University, Stanford, California

Contents

Foreword: Equity, Diversity, and Inclusion **xi**

Mark D. Miller

Preface: Equality, Diversity, and Inclusion in Sports Medicine **xiii**

Constance R. Chu, Erica Taylor, and Joel Boyd

Section I: Where we are

Trends for Diversity in Orthopedic Sports Medicine **213**

Pramod Kamalapathy, Laurel A. Barras, and David R. Diduch

Despite the increasingly diverse population of the United States, orthopedic surgery continues to lag other medical specialties in terms of diversity. It remains the specialty with the lowest percentage of women, and White physicians dominate the field, especially in leadership positions. Although the trends are slowly moving in the right direction, additional efforts must be taken to further diversify the field. A targeted, multifaceted approach is required to enhance awareness, educate, mentor, and develop future leaders. Such an approach has recently been established by the American Orthopaedic Society for Sports Medicine, which will hopefully improve future minority and female representation.

Gender Equity Efforts in Sports Medicine **221**

Emma E. Johnson, Gabriella E. Ode, Mary L. Ireland, Kellie Middleton, and Sommer Hammoud

Great progress has been made toward gender equality in athletics, whereas true equality has not yet been realized. Concurrently, women orthopedists along with advocate men have paved the way toward gender equity in orthopedics as a whole and more specifically in sports medicine. The barriers that contribute to gender disparities include lack of exposure, lack of mentorship, stunted career development, childbearing considerations and implicit gender bias and overt gender discrimination.

Racial and Ethnic Disparities in Sports Medicine and the Importance of Diversity **233**

Kellie K. Middleton and Alex Turner

Within orthopedics surgery as a specialty, sports medicine is one of the least diverse surgical subspecialties. Differences in minority representation between patient and provider populations are thought to contribute to disparities in care, access, and outcomes.

Section II: What can we do

Diversity in Orthopaedic Surgery: What Is Next? What is Needed Collectively? How Do You Go About Effecting Positive Change? **245**

Jason L. Koh

Orthopedic surgery as a field is the least diverse medical specialty. Multiple factors contribute to the lack of diversity, including lack of diversity in medical school, lack of role models and mentors, and discrimination and bias. Addressing the lack of diversity includes use of data, implementation of targeted pipeline programs, individual physician advocacy, institutional recruitment and DEI initiatives, and leadership from professional organizations. Targeted pipeline programs and role models and mentors are very effective in increasing diversity. Cultural change is occurring, and the future orthopaedic workforce will be more diverse.

Strengthening the Pipeline: Promoting Diversity into Orthopedic Surgery **253**

Maike van Niekerk, Alana O'Mara, Stephanie Kha, Joanne Zhou, Timothy A. McAdams, Amy Ladd, Kevin Shea, Steven Frick, William J. Maloney, and Constance R. Chu

The United States is a nation of diverse racial and ethnic origins. Athletes represent the full spectrum of the nation's population. However, the orthopedic surgeons who serve as team physicians are Caucasian and male with staggeringly few exceptions. This manuscript provides an overview of the current status and barriers to diversity among orthopedic team physicians, along with strategies to address the issue. Specifically, pipeline initiatives implemented at one academic medical school and orthopedic surgery department are summarized as potential models that can be further developed by other institutions to enhance diversity in orthopedic surgery.

Efforts to Improve Diversity, Equality, and Inclusion in Sports Medicine via Community Engagement Initiatives Within American Cities Divided by Racial, Social, and Economic Factors **271**

Michael D. Maloney, Ram Haddas, Edward M. Schwarz, Shaun Nelms, and Katherine Rizzone

Although the twenty-first century has seen major advances in evidence-based medicine to improve health, athletic performance, and injury prevention, our inability to implement these best practices across underserved American communities has limited the impact of these breakthroughs in sports medicine. Rochester, NY is stereotypical of American communities in which an economically challenged racially diverse urban center with grossly underperforming public schools is surrounded by adequately resourced predominantly Caucasian state-of-the-art education systems. As these great disparities perpetuate and further degrade our society in the absence of interventions, the need for community engagement initiatives is self-evident.

Sports Medicine Patient Experience: Implicit Bias Mitigation and Communication Strategies **279**

Pedro J. Tort Saadé and Augustus A. White III

Unconscious bias, also known as implicit bias, is the principal contributor to the perpetuation of discrimination and is a robust determinant of people's decision-making. Unconscious bias occurs despite conscious nonprejudiced intentions and interferes with the actions of the reflective and conscious side. Education and self-awareness about implicit bias and its potentially harmful effects on judgment and behavior may lead individuals to pursue corrective action and follow implicit bias mitigation communication strategies. Team physicians must follow existing communication strategies and guidelines to mitigate unconscious bias and begin an evolution toward nonbiased judgment and decision-making to improve athlete care.

Section III: Putting it together for a better future

The Intrinsic Value of Diversity in Team Leadership **293**

Chase Gauthier, Justin Kung, and Jeffrey Guy

Despite the demonstrated benefit of diversity within a team structure, there is a lack of diversity among leadership in professional organizations. An increase in diversity among leadership teams would allow for more effective communication with team members, better problem-solving skills, increased trust within a team environment, and greater inspiration for future generations. Therefore, diversity should be a core concept within a leadership team.

Diversity, Equity, and Inclusion Leadership: A True Team Sport **299**

Erica Taylor

The diversity, equity, and inclusion (DEI) leadership and team experience has evolved in response to a very dynamic state of change in our society and profession. In this review, the author has outlined *4* necessary components of empowering leaders and teams, including solidifying a common mission, creating value around the team and its purpose, measuring relevant and inclusive outputs, and cocreating a strategy that is meaningful and effectively achieves the true north. The author uses parallels from sports to define these pragmatic steps of a "DEI leaders' playbook" to move forward in the creation of healthy, inclusive environments.

Equality, Diversity, and Inclusion in Sports Medicine

CLINICS IN SPORTS MEDICINE

Foreword
Equity, Diversity, and Inclusion

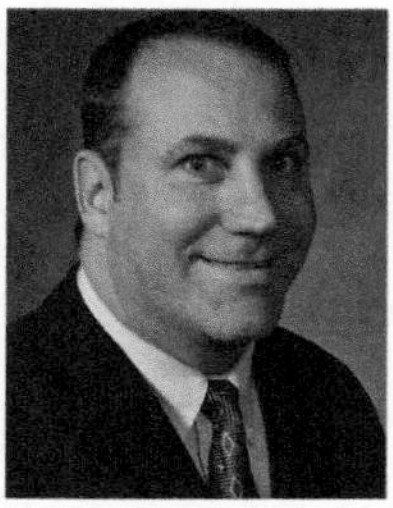

Mark D. Miller, MD, PE, Colonel USAF (Ret)
Consulting Editor

It is an honor and a pleasure to introduce this issue of *Clinics in Sports Medicine* entitled Equity, Diversity, and Inclusion in Sports Medicine. I have known and worked closely with Drs Chu and Taylor for over two decades. I sincerely thank them both for bringing this important topic to the attention of our readers, and in helping me better understand many of the concepts brought forth in this issue during my reign as President of the American Orthopaedic Society for Sports Medicine (AOSSM) last year. It is appropriate that this will be my last Foreword for *Clinics in Sports Medicine* as I turn over the privilege and responsibility as Consulting Editor to my junior colleague, Dr Winston Gwathmey. Please allow me to introduce this topic by paraphrasing a few thoughts from my AOSSM Presidential address:

Inclusion is an American Ideal and should be at the heart of all sports medicine organizations and individuals. It is simply a matter of recognition and acceptance—putting yourself in someone else's shoes. We should treat each other equally, regardless of race, gender, sexuality, or background. Jesse Jackson noted, "Inclusion is not a matter of political correctness. It is the key to growth." One might ask, "what is the difference between diversity and inclusion"? Verna Myers, an expert on this topic, provides a nice analogy: *Diversity is being invited to the party, Inclusion is being asked to dance.* So, let's dance!

Let's talk about Equity, Diversity, and Inclusion (DEI) more in-depth. First let's keep in mind the many types of diversity—race, sex/gender/sexual orientation, age, religion, culture, socioeconomic background, disability, and more. So, think for a minute—and even visualize—the diversity in these many categories, if you will, of places in your life: Your family and extended family, your clinics, your operating rooms, your department meetings, your places of worship, your golf clubs or gyms, your neighborhood. Some types of diversity may be obvious, and some may not. But I hope we can agree that diversity enriches us; it makes us better, more balanced, and more open to wider points of view. Those are good things. *Those are indeed good things.* My very

Clin Sports Med 43 (2024) xi–xii
https://doi.org/10.1016/j.csm.2024.01.002 sportsmed.theclinics.com

accomplished sister once told me (pejoratively, though with humor) that I was “male, pale, and stale.” Two of those things I can't do anything about, but one I can—let's truly embrace strategic ways to advance needed DEI initiatives to enrich who we are and what we do.

Racism is not always overt…in fact, there is a whole lexicon of terms for prejudice or bias. Inherent bias involves underlying assumptions; systemic bias is institutional, and implicit bias may be unintentional. The term "woke" simply means to be alert to racial prejudice and discrimination. You don't have to lean left to be woke!

With those concepts in mind, I am proud of the editors and contributors (many with connections, like me, to the University of Virginia and the Military) for an outstanding issue of *Clinics in Sports Medicine*. Let's all embrace Equity, Diversity, and Inclusion in our worlds. Thank you for allowing me to serve as Consulting Editor for this tremendous publication for the past 24 years!

Sincerely,

Mark D. Miller, MD, PE, Colonel USAF (Ret)
Division of Sports Medicine
Department of Orthopaedic Surgery
400 Ray C. Hunt Drive, Suite 330
Charlottesville, VA 22908-0159, USA

E-mail address:
MDM3P@hscmail.mcc.virginia.edu

Preface

Equality, Diversity, and Inclusion in Sports Medicine

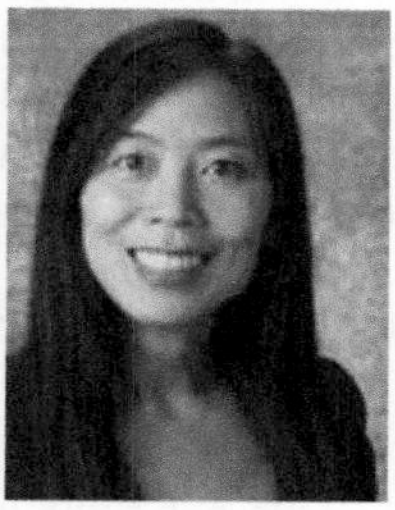
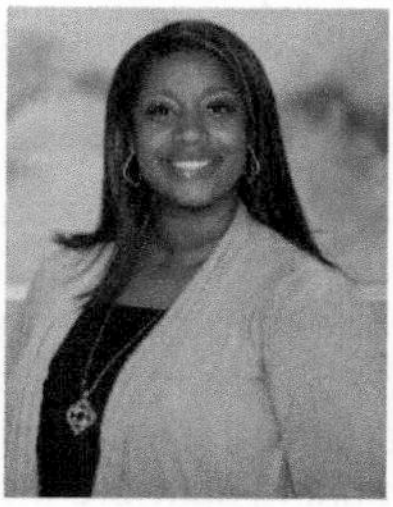
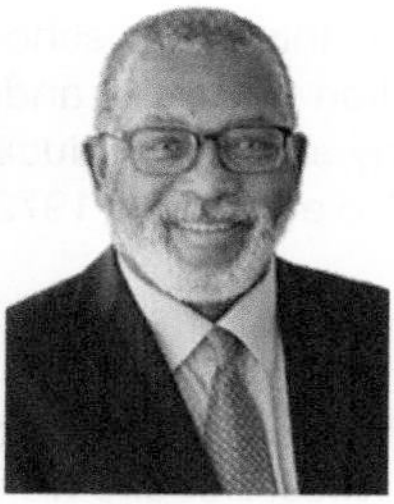

Constance R. Chu, MD   Erica Taylor, MD, MBA   Joel Boyd, MD
Editors

Sports offer a window into society far beyond the mechanics of participation. It can unite people across socioeconomic barriers with a common identity. Within the vast machinery of American sports, the distribution of power, roles, and opportunities often reflects that of historical norms within the broader society. While women and persons of color comprise a high percentage of athletes, representation is low in positions of influence where few serve as owners, consultants, coaches, athletic trainers, and team physicians. This special issue of *Clinics in Sports Medicine* highlights opportunities to embrace and enhance diversity, equity, and inclusion (DEI) among the medical teams that care for athletes.

Athletic prowess is widely celebrated, and sporting success has been a catalyst for change. The integration of professional sports preceded that of the military in 1948 and that of society after passage of the Civil Rights Act of 1964. The ideals of democracy that Americans of all races fought for in World War II clashed with the realities of Black oppression and Japanese internment back home. After World War II, there was growing pressure to integrate sports.[1] In 1946, the Los Angeles Rams signed Kenny Washington to play in the National Football League (NFL). An undisputed star at halfback for the UCLA Bruins, Washington won the 1939 Douglas Fairbanks trophy awarded to the nation's best college football player. Although Washington had suffered several knee injuries playing minor league football and was past his prime by 1946, he nevertheless broke the color barrier in professional football a year prior to

Clin Sports Med 43 (2024) xiii–xv
https://doi.org/10.1016/j.csm.2024.01.001
0278-5919/24/© 2024 Published by Elsevier Inc.

Jackie Robinson's historic start in baseball for the Brooklyn Dodgers in 1947. The National Basketball Association (NBA) was not far behind signing Black star players Chuck Cooper, Nat Clifton, and Earl Lloyd in the 1950 draft. Today, players of color are the majority in the NBA and the NFL.

As professional sports increased in prominence, caring for and returning injured athletes to competition rose in importance. The field of Sports Medicine gained ascendency in the 1960s, and the American Society for Sports Medicine (AOSSM) was formed in 1972. By this time, schools, colleges, and professional sports showed greater representation of Blacks and persons of color. Title IX prohibiting sex-based discrimination in any school or education program receiving funding from the federal government was also enacted in 1972 and heralded the expansion of girls and women in sports.

Today, more women and persons of color participate in sports at all levels. Yet, few team physicians come from these groups. Orthopedic surgeons, of which the vast majority are white men, play key roles in the care of athletes who suffer from musculoskeletal injuries at high rates. Despite women making up more than 50% of the population, the latest published census of the American Association of Orthopaedic Surgeons conducted in 2018 showed 5.8% responding as female orthopedic surgeons and other studies reporting as few as 1.5% African American orthopedic surgeons orthopedic surgeons.[2] Such discrepancies are highlighted in this issue along with strategies for mitigation.[2] The same census showed the racial/ethnic breakdown of orthopaedic surgeons to be nearly 85% Caucasian, 6.7% Asian, less than 2% African American, and .4% Native American.

At the highest levels of Orthopedic Sports Medicine, critical barriers have been broken. In 2021, Dr Clarence Shields became the first African American president of the AOSSM. Among persons of color, Dr Freddie Fu became the first foreign-born surgeon to assume Presidency of the AOSSM in 2008. In 2013, Dr Jo Hannafin became the first female President of AOSSM. Without question, there are innumerable trailblazers within Athletics and Sports Medicine who catalyzed advancement of DEI in various facets, serving as shouldering giants for all of us. These champions embody the true essence of perseverance, strength, and excellence.

We are experiencing an unprecedented level of awareness and attention to the persistent health disparities and societal injustices that are impacting our patients, loved ones, and teammates. Collectively, these realities implore us to address inequities effectively and with sincere intention. In recent years, the AOSSM has prioritized attention to DEI through the establishment of a Task Force, which became a standing Committee in 2023. Such emphasis on DEI has led to increased representation of diverse groups in Educational Programming as well as Committee and Leadership appointments. However, there is still much work to be done.

In this Special Edition issue, we invite you to explore the current state of DEI in Sports Medicine and incorporate the included expert advisement on how we can pave a path forward as One Team.

DISCLOSURES

C.R. Chu: Co-Chair of AOSSM DEI Committee. E. Taylor: Founder, Orthopaedic Diversity Leadership Consortium; Consultant: Johnson and Johnson DePuy Synthes; Speaker: Exactech. J. Boyd: I am an Arthrex Consultant.

Constance R. Chu, MD
Department of Orthopedic Surgery
Stanford University
Redwood City, CA 94063, USA

Erica Taylor, MD, MBA
Duke University School of Medicine
PO Box 1726
Wake Forest, NC 27587, USA

Joel Boyd, MD
TRIA Orthopedic Center
Bloomington, MN 55431, USA

E-mail addresses:
chucr@stanford.edu (C.R. Chu)
Erica.taylor@orthodiversity.org (E. Taylor)
Joel.Boyd@tria.com (J. Boyd)

REFERENCES

1. Farrell Evans. 9 Black Athletes Who Integrated Professional Sports. history.com. June 3, 2022.
2. 2AAOS. Orthopaedic Practice in the U.S. 2018.aaos.org. January 2019.

Section I: Where we are

Trends for Diversity in Orthopedic Sports Medicine

Pramod Kamalapathy, MD, Laurel A. Barras, MD,
David R. Diduch, MD*

KEYWORDS

• Orthopedics • Diversity • Race • Sex • Trends

KEY POINTS

- Orthopedic surgery continues to lag behind other specialties in terms of improving diversity.
- Foot and ankle, trauma, and sports medicine have the least diversity based on ethnicity of fellowship directors among the orthopedic subspecialties.
- The representation of female faculty based on the American Orthopaedic Society for Sports Medicine registry improved from 6% in 2015 to 9.5% in 2022; however, as of 2020, there was only one female fellowship director within orthopedic sports medicine.
- Although the diversity of sports medicine faculty is unknown, the majority (86%) of division chiefs have been reported to be White.
- Additional intentional efforts are needed to spread awareness, educate, and further hasten the improvement of minority representation in the field.

INTRODUCTION

The population in the United States is increasingly becoming more diverse and the importance of diversity in the workplace cannot be overstated. Numerous studies have found that diversity in the workplace increases employee morale, creates a wide range of perspectives to help solve difficult problems, and leads to better outcomes.[1,2] Specifically in health care, a lack of diversity can lead to limited perspectives, create implicit bias, contribute to poor care for the underserved, and propagate less diversity in future recruitment. Evidence suggests that heterogeneity can increase the cultural competence of the workforce and increase equitable treatment of patients.[2,3]

Within orthopedic literature, numerous studies have found that socioeconomic disparities play a large role in patient outcomes following surgery.[4,5] In fact, underrepresented minorities (URM) have decreased access and utilization of care compared

Department of Orthopaedic Surgery, University of Virginia, 1215 Lee Street, Charlottesville, VA 22903, USA

* Corresponding author. Department of Orthopaedic Surgery, UVA, P.O. Box 800159, Charlottesville, VA 22908.

E-mail address: DRD5C@uvahealth.org

Clin Sports Med 43 (2024) 213–219
https://doi.org/10.1016/j.csm.2023.06.009
sportsmed.theclinics.com

with White patients.[6] Although it is important to understand the intertwined cultural and systemic factors that affect the patient population, one modifiable factor is the diversity and inclusion among the health-care staff that serve the patients. Patients have reported feeling they can communicate better with providers that share similar cultural backgrounds.[7] Moreover, URM physicians treat a greater proportion of underinsured patients, leading to an increased patient satisfaction in underserved groups. To better serve and meet the needs of patients, the health-care system overall must match the diversity of the patient population.

It is imperative to highlight that orthopedic surgery continuously has one of the lowest percentages of women and minorities of all medical and surgical subspecialties.[8–13] In the 2020 to 2021 application cycle, medical school matriculants were 8.0% African American, 21.6% Asian, 6.9% Hispanic/Latino, 44.7% Caucasian, 53.7% women, and 46.3% men.[14] Meanwhile in 2020, the representation of women and minorities in orthopedic residency was 16.0% and 24.2%, respectively.[15] The present article will explore the current trends of diversity within orthopedic sports medicine.

Trends in Gender

To understand the demographics of orthopedic sports medicine, it is critical to analyze orthopedic surgery as a whole. Although women comprise greater than 50% of medical school graduates, orthopedic surgery remains the medical specialty with the lowest proportion of female residents at 14.0% in the 2016 to 2017 academic year—up from 11.0% in the 2005 to 2006 academic year.[9] This 27.3% increase during a 10 to 12-year period lags behind other male-dominated fields, such as neurological surgery (56.8%) and thoracic surgery (111.2%). Meanwhile, in 2020, the representation of women in orthopedic residency was only modestly improved to 16.0%.[15] Furthermore, residency programs have been training women at uneven rates. From 2014 to 2019, 37 residency programs had no female trainees, whereas 53 programs had more than 20% female trainees during at least one of those 5 years.[16]

Despite the numerous benefits, orthopedic surgery continues to slowly address gender parity. It is often cited that women encompass only 6.5% of members in the American Academy of Orthopaedic Surgeons (AAOS) database (**Fig. 1**).[17–19] Using a national provider identifier registry, Acuña and colleagues found that the percentage of female orthopedic surgeons increased from 6% in 2010 to 8% in 2020. Alarmingly, it was calculated that it would take more than 200 years to achieve gender parity in orthopedic surgery based on this trend.[20] Moreover, in the 2018 AAOS census, the average age of orthopedic surgeons was shown to increase from 50.7 in 2008 to 56.5 years. However, when analyzed based on gender, females comprised 15.9% of those aged younger than 40 years, whereas only 1.9% were aged older than 60 years, suggesting that there is reason to be optimistic regarding the future generation of surgeons in terms of gender parity.

Yet specifically within orthopedic sports medicine, 6% of faculty was female in 2015 based on American Orthopaedic Society for Sports Medicine (AOSSM) and 6.6% in 2017 based on the Association of American Medical Collections (AAMC). Currently, in 2022, there are 183 (9.5%) female sports medicine surgeons who are members of AOSSM. There may be an increase in representation of female faculty based on the latest distribution of graduating sports medicine fellows. Although the overall proportion of female sports fellows is encouraging with 10.9% in 2021, further investigation showed the distribution of sports medicine fellows has not changed significantly from 2016 (11.2%) to 2021 (10.9%). One reason for cautious optimism is that sports medicine is one of the more popular subspecialties among women.[18,21,22] In a survey

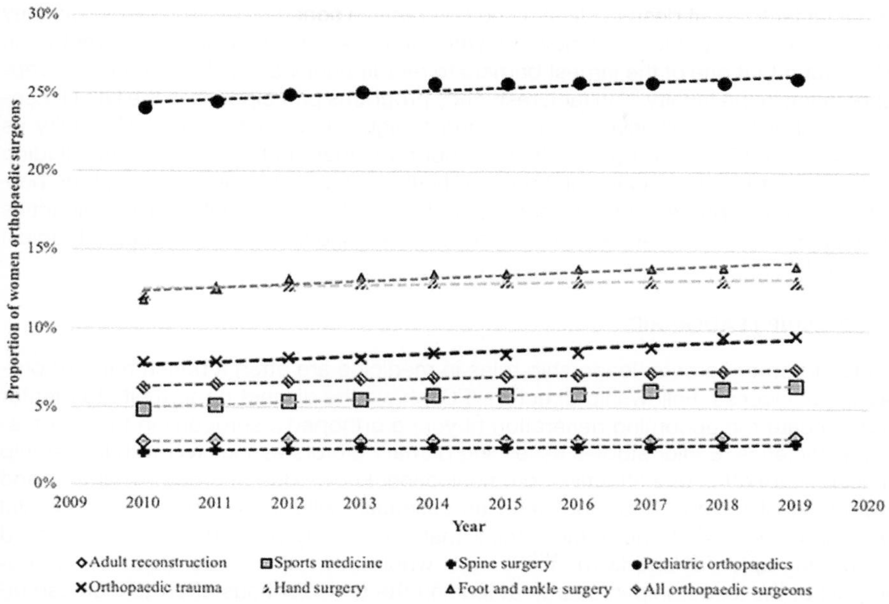

Fig. 1. Graph showing the proportion of women providers among orthopedic subspecialties. (Source: Acuña AJ, Sato EH, Jella TK et al. How Long Will It Take to Reach Gender Parity in Orthopaedic Surgery in the United States? An Analysis of the National Provider Identifier Registry. Clin Orthop Relat Res. 2021 Jun; 479(6): 1179–1189, Figure 3. Published online 2021 Mar 19. https://doi.org/10.1097/CORR.0000000000001724.)

of female orthopedic surgeons, the most common subspecialties in order were hand, pediatrics, and sports medicine, with a higher number of younger surgeons pursuing sports medicine.[21] In addition, various studies have shown that female orthopedic surgeons enter academia at a higher rate than men.[18,21,22]

Trends in Race

Not too long ago, the AAMC championed a campaign to enroll a medical school class containing at least 3000 students of color by the year 2000. Although the campaign did improve the overall numbers, it ultimately failed due to political backlash for admission based on the criteria of race. Medical schools have since continued to actively promote diversity among their incoming class to reflect the nation's diversity. In 2021, there was an increase in African American first-year students by 21% to 2562 students, which reflects a total of 11.3% of the entering medical school class population nationwide—up from 9.5% the previous year.[23]

Similarly, White physicians have predominated the workforce of orthopedic surgery. In the latest survey, the distribution of AAOS members showed that there were only 1.9% African Americans, 2.2% Hispanic/Latinos, and 6.7% Asian Americans.[24] Although the racial demographic of all sports medicine faculty is unknown, a recent study by Maqsoodi and colleagues[25] identified that division chiefs are largely 86% White, followed by Asian (11%), African American (1%), Hispanic/Latino (1%), and mixed ethnicity (1%).

Interestingly, Poon and colleagues[26] found that diversity decreased among orthopedic residents during a 10-year period from 2006 to 2015. This is possibly due to a variety of factors but despite URM being competitive academically for residency, they are entering orthopedic residency at lower rates.[27] A survey of program directors in 2020 found that one of the largest barriers to recruitment was the lack of minority representation in the faculty.[28] In fact, residency programs participating in the Nth Dimensions and/or Perry Initiative programs had a higher percentage of URM faculty as opposed to residency programs that did not participate in these programs, alluding to the impact that physicians of color can have on the culture and values of the program. Some improvements have been noted as the representation of minorities increased to around 24.2%, according to the Association of American Medical College.[15]

FELLOWSHIP LEADERSHIP

Similar to other careers, leadership roles in medicine are often a benchmark for professional success. Fellowship directors (FDs) have the distinct opportunity to mentor and educate the upcoming generation of young orthopedic surgeons in their professional societies. Earlier studies assessing primary factors associated with leadership in health care often cite effective communication, knowledge of group dynamics, and promotion of change and innovation as essential skills to becoming a successful physician leader.[29,30] The authors think that it is simply not enough to understand the demographic of sports medicine as a whole but rather understand the demographic of the leadership in charge of leading the conscientious effort to increase diversity among residents, fellows, and faculty.

A comparison of all fellowship director demographics in a study by Kamalapathy and colleagues[31] showed that sports medicine FDs have an average age of 54.5 ± 9.0 years. As of 2020, compared with all FDs in orthopedic surgery, the highest proportion of male FDs were in arthroplasty (100%, N = 94 men), sports medicine (98.9%, 87 men and 1 woman), and spine (96.1%, 99 men and 4 women).[31] Foot and ankle (n = 43, 89.6%), trauma (n = 53, 85.5%), and sports medicine (n = 75, 85.2%) had the least diversity based on ethnicity of FDs among all the orthopedic subspecialties. Specifically, in the sports medicine cohort, FDs were predominantly Caucasian (n = 75, 85.2%), followed by Asian American (n = 6, 6.8%), African American (n = 3, 3.4%), Middle Eastern (n = 3, 3.4%), and Hispanic/Latino (n = 1, 1.1%). This cross-sectional study revealed that there are disproportionately fewer women and minorities in fellowship director positions. A remarkable finding is that there is only 1 female surgeon in the role of FD within orthopedic sports medicine as of 2020.[31,32] Comparisons of the demographic distribution of sports medicine FDs appointed since 2015 and overall sports medicine FDs yielded no difference, demonstrating that perhaps other factors, such as research and institutional familiarity, were perceived to be more important.

FUTURE OUTLOOK

Targeted efforts have been made to promote diversity in orthopedic surgery. The Ruth Jackson Society (1983), Nth dimensions (2006), the Perry Initiative (2009), J. Robert Gladden Orthopaedic Society (1998), and the Women Orthopaedist Global Outreach (2006) are a few societies that aim to promote diversity in orthopedics to "increase the overall collective intelligence of the team."[33] The Forum Society of fellowship trained women orthopedic surgeons with practice interest in Sports Medicine provided fellowship within the field. Through active mentorship and career exposure, these societies continue to advocate for and aid underrepresented medical students and residents in their professional development. URM and women who attended a medical school at an institution with higher URM and female representation on the faculty and residency were more likely to apply to orthopedic surgery. However, more support and active mentorship is required to improve the diversity in orthopedic surgery.

Recently, AOSSM established the diversity initiative, which includes such programming as (1) an *AOSSM Diversity Task Force* that had evolved to a standing committee to engage all our leadership and programming to ensure the education of our membership on the issues of diversity, equality, and inclusion for the better of the athletes we serve; (2) *AOSSM Diversity Webinars* focused on educating our Emerging Leaders on this vitally important issue; (3) a *Diversity Education for Membership* as a key component of onboarding for all society members and leadership; and (4) an *AOSSM Pathways to Leadership* statement to educate all AOSSM members on how to become maximally involved in our society, and in doing so, become truly diverse.[34] Such a multifaceted approach to enhance awareness, educate regarding opportunities, mentor future surgeons, and develop future leaders is reason for optimism and something we all can support.

DISCLOSURE

The authors have no relevant disclosures.

FUNDING

There were no funding obtained for the study.

REFERENCES

1. Gomez LE, Bernet P. Diversity improves performance and outcomes. J Natl Med Assoc 2019;111(4):383–92.
2. Stanford FC. The importance of diversity and inclusion in the healthcare workforce. J Natl Med Assoc 2020;112(3):247–9.
3. Khuntia J, Ning X, Cascio W, et al. Valuing diversity and inclusion in health care to equip the workforce: survey study and pathway analysis. JMIR Form Res 2022; 6(5):e34808.
4. Paredes AZ, Hyer JM, Diaz A, et al. The impact of mental illness on postoperative outcomes among medicare beneficiaries: a missed opportunity to help surgical patients? Ann Surg 2020. https://doi.org/10.1097/SLA.0000000000004118.
5. Ali I, Vattigunta S, Jang JM, et al. Racial disparities are present in the timing of radiographic assessment and surgical treatment of hip fractures. Clin Orthop 2020;478(3):455–61.
6. Dunlop DD, Song J, Manheim LM, et al. Racial disparities in joint replacement use among older adults. Med Care 2003;41(2):288–98.
7. Association of Racial/Ethnic and Gender Concordance Between Patients and Physicians With Patient Experience Ratings | Health Disparities | JAMA Network Open | JAMA Network. Available at: https://jamanetwork.com/journals/jamanetworkopen/fullarticle/2772682?utm_source=For_The_Media&utm_medium=referral&utm_campaign=ftm_links&utm_term=110920. Accessed September 12, 2022.
8. Blakemore LC, Hall JM, Biermann JS. Women in surgical residency training programs. J Bone Joint Surg Am 2003;85(12):2477–80.
9. Chambers CC, Ihnow SB, Monroe EJ, et al. Women in orthopaedic surgery: population trends in trainees and practicing surgeons. J Bone Joint Surg Am 2018; 100(17):e116.

10. Day CS, Lage DE, Ahn CS. Diversity based on race, ethnicity, and sex between academic orthopaedic surgery and other specialties: a comparative study. J Bone Joint Surg Am 2010;92(13):2328–35.
11. Filiberto AC, Le CB, Loftus TJ, et al. Gender differences among surgical fellowship program directors. Surgery 2019;166(5):735–7.
12. Okike K, Utuk ME, White AA. Racial and ethnic diversity in orthopaedic surgery residency programs. J Bone Joint Surg Am 2011;93(18):e107.
13. Saxena S, Cannada LK, Weiss JM. Does the proportion of women in orthopaedic leadership roles reflect the gender composition of specialty societies? Clin Orthop 2020;478(7):1572–9.
14. 2020 FACTS: Applicants and Matriculants Data. AAMC. Available at: https://www.aamc.org/data-reports/students-residents/interactive-data/2020-facts-applicants-and-matriculants-data. Accessed January 19, 2021.
15. Report on Residents. AAMC. Available at: https://www.aamc.org/data-reports/students-residents/report/report-residents. Accessed January 22, 2021.
16. Van Heest AE, Agel J. The uneven distribution of women in orthopaedic surgery resident training programs in the United States. J Bone Joint Surg Am 2012; 94(2):e9.
17. Cvetanovich GL, Saltzman BM, Chalmers PN, et al. Research productivity of sports medicine fellowship faculty. Orthop J Sports Med 2016;4(12). https://doi.org/10.1177/2325967116679393.
18. O'Reilly OC, Day MA, Cates WT, et al. Female team physician representation in professional and collegiate athletics. Am J Sports Med 2020;48(3):739–43.
19. Research Resources - American Academy of Orthopaedic Surgeons. Available at: https://www.aaos.org/quality/research-resources/Accessed January 11, 2021.
20. Acuña AJ, Sato EH, Jella TK, et al. How long will it take to reach gender parity in orthopaedic surgery in the United States? An analysis of the national provider identifier registry. Clin Orthop 2021;479(6):1179–89.
21. Bratescu RA, Gardner SS, Jones JM, et al. Which subspecialties do female orthopaedic surgeons choose and why? JAAOS Glob Res Rev 2020;4(1). https://doi.org/10.5435/JAAOSGlobal-D-19-00140.
22. Rynecki ND, Krell ES, Potter JS, et al. How well represented are women orthopaedic surgeons and residents on major orthopaedic editorial boards and publications? Clin Orthop 2020;478(7):1563–8.
23. Medical School Enrollment More Diverse in 2021. AAMC. Available at: https://www.aamc.org/news-insights/press-releases/medical-school-enrollment-more-diverse-2021. Accessed September 14, 2022.
24. AAOS Now September 2019: A Snapshot of U.S. Orthopaedic Surgeons: Results from the 2018 OPUS Survey. Available at: https://www.aaos.org/aaosnow/2019/sep/youraaos/youraaos01/. Accessed January 11, 2021.
25. Maqsoodi N, Mesfin A, Li X. Academic, leadership, and demographic characteristics of orthopaedic sports medicine division chiefs in the United States. JAAOS Glob Res Rev 2022;6(1):e21, 00139.
26. Poon S, Kiridly D, Mutawakkil M, et al. Current trends in sex, race, and ethnic diversity in orthopaedic surgery residency. J Am Acad Orthop Surg 2019;27(16): e725–33.
27. Poon S, Nellans K, Rothman A, et al. Underrepresented minority applicants are competitive for orthopaedic surgery residency programs, but enter residency at lower rates. J Am Acad Orthop Surg 2019;27(21):e957.
28. McDonald TC, Drake LC, Replogle WH, et al. Barriers to increasing diversity in orthopaedics. JBJS Open Access 2020;5(2):e0007.

29. Mrkonjic L, Grondin SC. Introduction to concepts in leadership for the surgeon. Thorac Surg Clin 2011;21(3):323–31.
30. Stone JL, Aveling EL, Frean M, et al. Effective leadership of surgical teams: a mixed methods study of surgeon behaviors and functions. Ann Thorac Surg 2017;104(2):530–7.
31. Kamalapathy P, Raso J, Rahman R, et al. Orthopaedic surgery fellowship directors: trends in demographics, education, employment, and institutional familiarity. HSS J 2023;19(1):113–9.
32. Kamalapathy P, Moore A, Brockmeier S, et al. Status quo: trends in diversity and unique traits among orthopaedic sports medicine fellowship directors. J Am Acad Orthop Surg 2022;30(1):36–43.
33. Day MA, Owens JM, Caldwell LS. Breaking barriers: a brief overview of diversity in orthopedic surgery. Iowa Orthop J 2019;39(1):1–5.
34. AOSSM Board of Directors Unanimously Approves Society's Diversity and Inclusion Program. Available at: https://www.newswise.com/articles/aossm-board-of-directors-unanimously-approves-society-s-diversity-and-inclusion-program. Accessed September 20, 2022.

Gender Equity Efforts in Sports Medicine

Emma E. Johnson, MD[a], Gabriella E. Ode, MD[b],
Mary L. Ireland, MD[c], Kellie Middleton, MD[d],
Sommer Hammoud, MD[a,*]

KEYWORDS

• Gender disparity • Mentorship • Childbearing consideration

KEY POINTS

- The stark gender disparities still remain in sports medicine, especially in department leadership roles, team physician roles, and research.
- The barriers that contribute to these disparities including lack of exposure, lack of mentorship, stunted career development, childbearing considerations and implicit gender bias and overt gender discrimination.
- Groups such as AOSSM, AAOS, RJOS, and Nth dimensions have established avenues for early exposure and mentorship facilitation, but more progress is needed.

GENDER DISPARITY IN ORTHOPEDIC SURGERY

According to the 2021 Association of American Medical Colleges (AAMC) matriculant data, 56% of medical students are women but there remains a clear lack of representation of women among all surgical specialties.[1–6] Specifically, the success of gender equity efforts in orthopedics has significantly lagged behind all other surgical specialties.[7,8] The most recent literature reports that 16.7% of orthopedic residents are women and 7.6% of practicing orthopedic surgeons are women.[9,10] Further, women orthopedic surgeons are concentrated in certain metropolitan areas in the Northwest, West, Northeast, and Southwest areas of the United States, with relatively little gender diversity among orthopedic surgeons in Midwestern and Southern states.[11] The current rate of gender diversification was reported using a compounded annual growth rate of 2% from 2010 to 2019.[12] At this rate, Acuña and colleagues predicted gender parity with the overall medical profession, which is currently 36.3% women, would not occur until 2236. Furthermore, it would not be until 2354 to achieve gender parity with the overall US population which is currently 50.8% women.[12]

[a] Rothman Orthopaedic Institute, Philadelphia, PA, USA; [b] Department of Orthopaedics, Hospital for Special Surgery, New York, NY, USA; [c] University of Kentucky, Lexington, KY, USA; [d] Northside Hospital Orthopaedic Institute, Lawrenceville, GA, USA
* Corresponding author.
E-mail address: Sommer.Hammoud@rothmanortho.com

Clin Sports Med 43 (2024) 221–232
https://doi.org/10.1016/j.csm.2023.06.020
0278-5919/24/

Gender Disparity in Sports Medicine

In a 2019 survey, the highest percentage of women orthopedic residents choose to subspecialize after residency in hand surgery (24.0%), pediatric orthopedics (22.6%), and sports medicine (16.3%).[13] Based on the SF Match fellowship data from 2010 to 2014, the greatest absolute numbers of women pursued sports medicine (94 women overall).[14] Although sports medicine is one of the most popular subspecialties for women to specialize in, gender disparities still remain prominent within this field. The AAMC reported in 2017 that 6.6% of sports medicine orthopedic surgeons were women.[15]

A benchmark for professional success in medicine is promotion to leadership roles. The role of fellowship director is considered a leadership position within an academic orthopedic department. The objective criteria to become a sports medicine fellowship program director include completion of an Accreditation Council for Graduate Medical Education's (ACGME)-accredited orthopedic sports medicine fellowship, at least 3 years of clinical practice, 3 years as a faculty member in an ACGME-accredited or Alpha Omega Alpha-approved orthopedic surgery and/or fellowship program, and certification in the subspecialty for which they are appointed as fellowship director. Belk and colleagues reported that currently there were 3/90 (3.3%) women orthopedic sports medicine fellowship directors for the 2020 to 2021 academic year.[16] This is an increase from the previous year, during which Kamalapathy and colleagues reported only one fellowship director was a woman.[17,18] These figures are staggering, especially in the context of the overall trends demonstrated in the national rates of women in orthopedic academic faculty positions. Shah and colleagues found that in 2017, women occupied 17.9% of orthopedic academic faculty positions.[19] Although this figure is promising compared with the overall proportion of women practicing orthopedic surgeons, which is closer to 7%, the growth rate of the proportion of women orthopedic surgeons in senior faculty appointments was significantly slower than other specialties over 20 years (7.3% vs 14.7%; $P < .001$).[19]

The role of subspecialty chief and department chair in orthopedic surgery is another critical departmental leadership role. Of the 191 orthopedic residency programs identified by Maqsoodi and colleagues, 100 programs had a sports medicine subspecialty division led by a division chief, and 96% of those division chiefs were men.[20] In 2019, Peck and colleagues reported that one of 119 orthopedic chairs were women, amounting to less than 1%. Furthermore, they found that the semantics used by orthopedic program to describe departmental leaders were less progressive than other specialties, with 71/119 (60%) of orthopedic department Web sites using the term "chairman" rather than the gender neutral term of "chair."[21]

Gender Disparity Among Team Physicians

In orthopedic sports medicine, the role of the team physician carries importance both from a leadership perspective as well as for achieving representation of the athlete–patients. Based on the publicly available sex-related data on select National Collegiate Athletics Association (NCAA) Division I collegiate athletes and professional sports organizations in 2020, 12.7% (112/879) of all team physicians were women.[22] However, only 26.8% (30/112) of these women team physicians were orthopedic surgeons. On the professional level, 6.3% of orthopedic surgeon team physicians were women. The professional organization with the highest proportion of women orthopedic surgeon physicians was found to be in the Women's National Basketball Association at 31.3%.[22] In contrast, in the National Basketball League (NBA) from 2009 to 2019, Hinkle and colleagues found that only 3 of 125 (2.4%) of team physicians were women.[23]

Wiggins and colleagues conversely examined the NBA, Major League Soccer, National Football League (NFL), National Hockey League, and Major League Baseball based on their high viewership and visibility. Of the 155 head team physicians identified, only 6 were women (3.9%).[24] Given how instrumental early exposure to orthopedics has been to encouraging women interest in orthopedics, increasing the number of team physicians on such widely televised teams may help introduce more young women to the possibilities available through orthopedic surgery. Furthermore, increasing the number of women team physicians may help decrease any implicit gender bias in treating women athletes.

Gender Disparity in Research

Academic productivity is an important requisite for each level of orthopedic training as well as promotion thereafter. In examining the academic productivity of women in sports medicine over a 46-year period, Kim and colleagues found that the proportion of women authors increased from 2.6% (1972–1979) to 14.7% (2010–2018) across *American Journal of Sports Medicine (AJSM), Arthroscopy, Journal of Shoulder and Elbow Surgery (JSES), and Sports Health.*[25] However, women authors averaged fewer publications than men and were more likely to be attributed middle authorship than senior authorship.[25] Women authors were also more likely to be full-time researchers such as PhD scientists as opposed to practicing clinicians.[25] Through further analysis of authors with mature research careers of 20 years or more, they found that women were most likely to hold middle authorship positions throughout their publication history. In contrast, men transitioned from writing mostly first-author publications in the first quartile of publication to senior author positions in their third and fourth quartiles. Moreover, the top publishing women produced 3.4 times fewer publications than male authors, despite a greater percentage of them being full-time research personnel. The results of this study align with prior reports that women have lower H-indices and align with publishing trends in orthopedics as a whole.

Rynecki and colleagues examined the gender composition of editorial boards and of first and last authors in The Journal of Bone and Joint Surgery (JBJS), The Journal of the American Academy of Orthopedic Surgeons (AAOS), and Clinical Orthopedics and Related Research (CORR) at three time points, with the most recent being 2017. They found in 2017 that 723/5391 (13%) of first or last authors were women, and 10/107 (9%) editors were women. Furthermore, there were no women editor-in-chiefs.[26] A similar study performed by Hiller and colleagues examined JBJS, CORR, and AJSM from 2006 to 2017. Across the study period, the investigators found that only 12% (211/1697) of first authors in AJSM were women, although this represented a 64% increase in representation of first author women.[27] Another study by Brown and colleagues looked at the representation of women in orthopedic research in different subspecialties in JBJS, AJSM, Journal of Arthroplasty, Journal of Orthopedic Trauma, Journal of Hand Surgery, and Journal of Pediatric Orthopedics from 1987 to 2017. Over this period, although there was an increase in the proportion of women first authors of academic orthopedic publications commensurate with expectations, the increase in proportion of women senior authors over that same study period was lower than expected. Furthermore, the increase in senior authorship was outpaced by both the increase in women residents and in women attending orthopedic surgeons.[28]

Participation at national conferences has also demonstrated a significant gender disparity. When examining participation of women orthopedic surgeons as moderators or course instructors at American Orthopedic Society of Sports Medicine (AOSSM) over a 5-year period from 2015 to 2019, Potter and colleagues found that an average of 6.7% of moderators and course instructors was women.[29] This figure reflects a growth from 6.3% in 2015 to 7.7% in 2019.[29] This proportion is in line with the 6.7% of women sports medicine physicians, reported by the AAMC in 2017[15] but remains less than for orthopedics as a whole. When evaluating women participation across all orthopedic subspecialties, Gerull and colleagues found that 535/3928 (14%) of annual meeting speakers across 19 national orthopedic societies were women, which was proportional to the 4389/33,051 (13%) of society members who were women according to 2018 data.[30]

HOW REPRESENTATION AFFECTS PATIENT CARE

Because the advent of Title IX just over 50 years ago, participation of women in organized sports has increased tremendously at all levels, including high school, collegiate, and professional levels. In fact, the number of females playing competitive sports in high school increased from less than 300,000 before the passing of Title IX to over 3.4 million in 2017 to 2018, a growth rate of 1033%.[31] As the number of women athletes continues to increase, the sex-related differences in prevalence and outcomes of many sports-related injuries have become increasingly more apparent.[32,33] Women athletes are up to 10 times more likely to sustain an anterior cruciate ligament (ACL) tear.[34–36] Women also sustain more concussions than men in gender-comparable sports and suffer greater memory deficits following concussions.[37,38] Patellar instability has been demonstrated to be more common in women, along with atraumatic multidirectional shoulder instability, ankle sprains and chronic ankle instability, and stress fractures.[33,36,39,40]

With the increase in awareness of sex-based differences in orthopedics and specifically sports medicine, there has been an increase in Women Sports Medicine Programs, which specialize in treating sports medicine conditions in women. In 2019, Hayes and colleagues identified 19 programs, with the majority being founded within the last 6 to 10 years.[41] These programs typically consist of a multidisciplinary team including orthopedic sports medicine, primary care sports medicine, athletic trainers, physical therapy, and in more expansive groups can also include general internal medicine, endocrinology, maternal fetal medicine, psychiatry, and musculoskeletal radiology.[42] These centers are most frequently led by women orthopedic surgeons. Unsurprisingly, several research studies have shown that women researchers are more likely to study research participants that were women rather than men.[43,44] Thus, increasing female representation in sports medicine will likely bolster the investigation and care of sex-specific differences in the sports medicine patient population.

BARRIERS TO WOMEN: LACK OF EXPOSURE

One of the reasons attributed to the low interest of women pursuing orthopedics is lack of exposure, particularly in medical school.[45–47] Baldwin and colleagues found that younger age, personal, independent, and school exposures to the field were significantly related to interest in orthopedics among women students.[45] This is echoed by the findings of Bernstein and colleagues who found that required instruction in musculoskeletal medicine was associated with a 12% higher rate of application to orthopedic surgery residency programs among students. This difference was more pronounced among women at a 75% difference in rate of application between those who had versus had not received required instruction in musculoskeletal medicine.[48] Rahman and colleagues surveyed 131 students from 27 medical students before and after an orthopedic clinical rotation and found that underrepresented minority and women student's overall perceptions of orthopedics significantly improved after doing a clinical rotation in proportion to the inclusiveness, friendliness, and diverse representation present in orthopedics. Despite significant improvement between pre-rotation and post-rotation ratings, their ratings on a scale from 1 to 5 remained below 2, and was negatively affected by low diversity and inclusion within orthopedics and overall perception of sexist behavior witnessed in the field.[49]

Exposure before medical school may also play a very important role. Johnson and colleagues surveyed 622 fourth year medical students with 125 entering orthopedics, and 497 that were not. Although the career choice in both groups was most influenced by third and fourth year clinical rotations and faculty relationships, those entering orthopedics were more likely than non-orthopedic bound medical students to be influenced by experiences and people before medical school.[50] Bernstein and colleagues also found that the impact of orthopedic exposure before medical was more influential in applicant men.[48]

The Ruth Jackson Orthopedic Society, the Forum, The Perry Initiative, and the Nth Dimension offer programs geared toward garnering interest and providing mentorship opportunities starting in high school, targeting both women and minorities.[51] Since its inception in 2009, The Perry Initiative has reached a total of over 12,000 students and now hosts 70 programs annually including 45 programs for high school women and 25 programs for women in medical school. Although the path from high school to residency is at minimum 9 to 12 years, the preliminary data demonstrate that the match rate for women who previously attended Perry Initiative programming is 20%.[52] This is higher than the current percentage of women in orthopedic residencies. When looking at the more immediate impact of Perry Initiative programs on perceptions, following the Perry Initiative Outreach Program and Medical Student Outreach Program at the University of Alabama at Birmingham Campus, Coffin and colleagues found that the program improved perceptions of both high school and medical students. In particular, participants had more positive perceptions regarding a woman orthopedist's ability to have work–life balance, family life, and children during orthopedics residency. Participation in the Perry Initiative event increased average interest in orthopedics by 28% among high school and 11% among medical school students.[53] On a larger scale, the survey responses collected from 206 participants who participated in medical student outreach program (MSOP) programs from 2012 to 2014 mirrored these improvements. These survey results demonstrated positive shifts in participants' perceptions regarding lifestyle, workforce diversity, length of training, physical demands, and competitiveness following the event, compared with pre-event survey responses.[54] The AAOS Nth Dimensions Summer Internship Program has had similar success. In data published in 2016, 31% (9/29) of the women who participated in the program applied for orthopedic surgery, which is significantly higher than the 1% who apply nationally.[55]

The continued expansion of these programs is an important element to increase early exposure to orthopedics. Regarding exposure to sports medicine, the NFL has started a clinical rotation program to promote sports medicine exposure to minority medical students from historically black colleges and universities. We would urge other national leagues to consider similar, yet expanded intersectional pipeline approaches to promote sports medicine exposure for both women and underrepresented minorities.

Barriers to Women: Lack of Mentorship

Another recognized barrier inhibiting women from entering orthopedics is the lack of woman to woman mentorship. Jagsi and colleagues reported that women medical students were more likely to enter programs with higher rates of women residents, reinforcing that same-gender mentors in both residents and faculty members may be important in recruiting women into orthopedics.[56] This is reiterated by the study by Okike and colleagues who found that of the 22,707 women who graduated from medical school from 2015 to 2017, 449 of the applied to an orthopedic surgery residency program. Of those women, those who attended medical school at institutions with high gender diversity among faculty were more likely to apply into orthopedics (OR = 1.3; $P = .023$). Similarly, women who attended medical school at institutions with high orthopedic resident gender diversity were more likely to apply into orthopedics (OR = 1.3; $P = .019$).[57] Organizations, such as Nth Dimension, the Perry Initiative and Ruth Jackson Society, provide opportunities for prospective applicants to meet potential mentors. Although the same gender mentors are clearly important, there is a need for more men orthopedic surgeons to step into mentorship roles and serve as advocates for women entering orthopedic surgery. Programming geared toward this at national meetings such as AAOS and AOSSM have recently served as a promising first step. In 2016, Samara Friedman created the "Women in Orthopedics" Facebook group with 400 initial members, which has now grown to more than 1500 members. This group serves as a safe space to share experiences, ask clinical questions, network, and support each other.[58]

Barriers to Women: Stunted Career Development

With few women faculty members in program director, department chair, and division chair positions, orthopedic surgery is often seen to have a glass ceiling. As residency programs focus to recruit more women into their programs, they should also consider addressing challenges to recruiting and promoting more women faculty.

One additional obstacle to career development among women in orthopedics involves compensation. Robin and colleagues reviewed the Centers for Medicare and Medicaid Services payments from each of the 10 largest orthopedic companies from 2013 to 2017 to identify demographic factors of orthopedic surgeons with the highest compensation. Among 347 orthopedic surgeons identified to have the highest compensation, only one surgeon was a woman (0.29%). The top 25 earners were composed of spine (32.9%), adult reconstruction (27.9%), and sports medicine (14.5%) subspecialists. Furthermore, sports medicine orthopedic surgeons had a significantly higher total mean payment amounts in comparison to all other specialties.[59] This was further corroborated by the work of Buerba and colleagues who found that of the 22,307 surgeons included in their analysis of Physician Payments Sunshine Act Web site, women ($n = 1298$) received smaller research and non-research payments than men, despite a greater proportion of them being in academics.[60] One possible explanation for this was that a greater proportion of women were in specialties that receive lower industry payments, such as foot and ankle, hand, and pediatrics. However, when they adjusted for academic rank and subspecialty using multivariable regressions, they found women still receive smaller industry payments compared with men.

Barriers to Women: Childbearing Considerations

One of the concerns medical students considering orthopedic surgery note is the lack of work–life balance.[45] Encompassed in the implications of work–life balance for women is childbearing considerations. Poon and colleagues surveyed 801 women orthopedic surgeons regarding fertility, pregnancy, and childbearing.[61] The average maternal age at first childbirth was 33.6 ± 3.6 years. Of those with children, 53% (425/801) reported childbearing was intentionally delayed due to their career choice. Twenty-four percent of the orthopedists reported that they had complications during their pregnancy. The trends of these findings were also reflected in the findings of Hamilton and colleagues who surveyed 223 orthopedic surgeons in comparison to eight other surgical specialties.[62] The percentage of orthopedic respondents who had at least one child during residency was comparable to respondents from other specialties (56/223 or 25.1% orthopedic surgeons vs 215/798 or 26.9%). To explore the sentiments of current residents regarding childbearing considerations, Mulcahey and colleagues surveyed 190 women residents. Most (83.7%) of the residents reported that they did not have children during residency and were not pregnant at the time of survey. Forty-eight percent of respondents reported that they had deferred having children because they were in residency. Regarding the culture around having children in residency, 59.5% of women residents reported that they had experienced bias from co-residents and 49.5% had experienced bias from attendings regarding women having children during residency. Reid and colleagues also found that women residents were more likely to report delaying having children during residency (56.7% vs 38.7%; $P = .001$).[63] Women residents were also more likely than men to cite reputational concerns (57.6% vs 0.7%; $P < .001$) and effects on career opportunities (42.4% vs 7.6%; $P < .001$) as reasons for delaying parenthood.

These concerns are further supported by the perceptions of pregnancy and parenthood during orthopedic surgery residency by program directors, investigated by Nemeth and colleagues.[64] Fifty-three percent (26/49) of program directors who were men believed pregnancy and parenthood negatively affected women residents' scholarly activities, whereas 83% (10/12) of women program directors believed it had no effect. Further, significantly more program directors reported believing that women resident pregnancy and parenthood imposed a greater burden on co-residents than parenthood for men residents (77% vs 45.9%).

Beyond just the perceptions of residents and faculty, the logistics of maternity leave are also prohibitory at some programs. In 2016, it was found that only 55% of orthopedic programs offered parental leave beyond the regular annual vacation time.[65] The American Board of Orthopaedic Surgeons (ABOS) has recently allowed for maternity leave without requiring additional time added onto the overall duration of residency by adjusting the requirements to 46 weeks of orthopedic education per year, averaged over 5 years.[66] One additional concern is that even after residency training concludes, taking maternity leave means time off without seeing patients during the trial period for tenure. Some have suggested extending the time to reach tenure or stopping the clock during maternity leave to foster an environment for women surgeons to reach full professorship while balancing family obligations.

Barriers to Women: Implicit Bias and Overt Discrimination

Prior research has indicated that the drop-off in women representation from medical school to orthopedic residency does not occur during the application process itself. Scherl and colleagues investigated the initial residency application review process by creating a copy of each of the women applicants and altering the gender and name and then comparing the rankings of several reviews to determine if gender played any role in ranking. They found no evidence of bias against women applicants in the initial application review phase ($P = .5$). Further, Day and colleagues found that the women representation among applicants paralleled their representation among orthopedic residents. This is not to say that the application process is without bias. Hern and colleagues found that in residency interviews of all applicants, women are more likely to be asked prohibited questions during residency interviews. These questions included questions about marital status, parental status, and plans for childbearing. Overall, those who were asked about gender or childbearing plans tended to rank programs lower because of those questions. Further, the frequency of being asked inappropriate interview questions was higher in orthopedics at 84.7% than any other specialty other than neurosurgery (86.0%).[67] In a survey looking at orthopedic applicants specifically,

Huntington and colleagues found that women were asked significantly more gender-related questions than men during their interview (57.1% vs 5.3%; $P < .001$). In this same study, they found that applicant men were significantly less likely than women applicants to agree with the statement "the field of orthopedics needs more women orthopaedists" ($P < .001$).[68]

Of the 927 members of the AAOS surveyed, 66% of members reported experiencing discrimination, harassment, bullying, or sexual harassment in their careers, 81% of which were women. Specifically, 84% of women experienced discrimination compared with 59% of men ($P < .05$). Fifty-four percent of women experienced sexual harassment compared with 10% of men ($P < .05$).[69] Whicker and colleagues looked at the prevalence of sexual harassment during residency training specifically and of the 250 women orthopedic surgeons surveyed, 68% reported having experienced sexual harassment during their orthopedic training.[70] Of these women, only 7% reported this harassment to their program director and only 5% to an attending surgeon. The main deterrents to why they did not report included negative impact on career (50%), a belief that reporting would be pointless because the department would not take action (43%) and not wanting to report a superior (39%).

The efforts of "Speak Up Ortho" have brought to light some of the shocking and atrocious stories of harassment and discrimination against women orthopedic physicians in the workplace.[71] Fear of retaliation and detriment to one's career are two common reasons for lack of reporting and filing complaints about these behaviors. Cannada and colleagues outline important ways to improve culture and mitigate harassment. These include (1) developing a process to report harassment concerns without fear of retaliation and (2) building a consistent vetting process for applicants for positions in all aspects of orthopedics regarding their commitment to diversity, equity, and inclusion. Such positions would include faculty candidates, program directors, department chairs, board examiners, and AAOS Board of Director positions. (3) Training people on how to have uncomfortable, but essential conversations, particularly those related to perceptions of harassment and micro-aggressions, and (4) including the mandatory teaching of bystander intervention to all trainees and faculty in residency programs.[58]

SUMMARY AND FUTURE STEPS

As we celebrate 50 years since the enactment of title IX, we recognize that great progress has been made toward gender equality in athletics, whereas true equality has not yet been realized. Concurrently, women orthopedists along with advocate men have paved the way toward gender equity in orthopedics as a whole and more specifically in sports medicine. However, this article highlights the stark gender disparities that still remain in sports medicine, especially in department leadership roles, team physician roles, and research. We highlight the barriers that contribute to these disparities including lack of exposure, lack of mentorship, stunted career development, and childbearing considerations, and implicit gender bias and overt gender discrimination.

We hope that societies such as Ruth Jackson Orthopedic Society, the Forum, The Perry Initiative, Nth Dimensions, AOSSM, and AAOS will continue to lead orthopedics toward addressing gender disparities that remain pervasive. We encourage our readers to get involved in these efforts.

DISCLOSURE

Emma Johnson: No relevant disclosures. Gabriella Ode: American Orthopaedic Association (board or comittee member), American Shoulder and Elbow Surgerons (board or committee member), Arthroscopy Asssociation of North America (board or committee member) Exactech, Inc (paid presenter or speaker). Mary Ireland: AAOS (board or commitee member), American college of sports medicine (board or committee member), AOSSM (board or committee member), female athlete triad coalition (board or committee member), Orthopaedic Research and Education Foundation (board or committee member), Smith & Nephew (paid presenter), UpToDate (publishing royalies, financial or material support). Kellie Middleton: Smith & Nephew (employee), Stryker (paid consult). Sommer Hammoud: AOSSM (board or committee member), Arthrex (paid consult), Orthopaedic Learning Center (board or committee member), Perry Initiative (board or committee member).

REFERENCES

1. Jonasson O. Leaders in American surgery: where are the women? Surgery 2002; 131(6):672–5.
2. Seemann NM, Webster F, Holden HA, et al. Women in academic surgery: why is the playing field still not level? Am J Surg 2016;211(2):343–9.
3. Sexton KW, Hocking KM, Wise E, et al. Women in academic surgery: the pipeline is busted. J Surg Educ 2012;69(1):84–90.
4. Weiss A, Lee KC, Tapia V, et al. Equity in surgical leadership for women: more work to do. Am J Surg 2014;208(3):494–8.
5. Zhuge Y, Kaufman J, Simeone DM, et al. Is there still a glass ceiling for women in academic surgery? Ann Surg 2011;253(4):637–43.
6. Association of American Medical Colleges. Table A-7.2: Applicants, First-Time Applicants, Acceptees, and Matriculants to U.S. Medical Schools by Sex, 2011-2012 through 2020-2021.; 2020. Available at: https://www.aamc.org/system/files/2020-10/2020_FACTS_Table_A-7.2.pdf. Accessed October 1, 2022.
7. Blakemore LC, Hall JM, Biermann JS. Women in surgical residency training programs. J Bone Joint Surg Am 2003;85(12):2477–80.
8. Rohde RS, Wolf JM, Adams JE. Where Are the Women in Orthopaedic Surgery? Clin Orthop Relat Res 2016;474(9):1950–6.
9. Accreditation Council for Graduate Medical Education. ACGME Data Resource Book.; 2020. Available at: http://www.acgme.org/About-Us/Publications-and-Resources/Graduate-Medical-Education-Data-Resource-Book. Accessed September 18, 2022.
10. Cherf J. A snapshot of U.S. orthopaedic surgeons: results from the 2018 OPUS survey. AAOS Now. Available at: https://www.aaos.org/aaosnow/2019/sep/youraaos/youraaos01/. Published September 2019. Accessed October 1, 2022.
11. Peterman NJ, Macinnis B, Stauffer K, et al. Gender Representation in Orthopaedic Surgery: A Geospatial Analysis From 2015 to 2022. Cureus 2022;14(7): e27305.
12. Acuña AJ, Sato EH, Jella TK, et al. How Long Will It Take to Reach Gender Parity in Orthopaedic Surgery in the United States? An Analysis of the National Provider Identifier Registry. Clin Orthop Relat Res 2021;479(6):1179–89.
13. Bratescu RA, Gardner SS, Jones JM, et al. Which Subspecialties Do Female Orthopaedic Surgeons Choose and Why?: Identifying the Role of Mentorship and Additional Factors in Subspecialty Choice. J Am Acad Orthop Surg Glob Res Rev 2020;4(1):e1900140.
14. Cannada LK. Women in Orthopaedic Fellowships: What Is Their Match Rate, and What Specialties Do They Choose? Clin Orthop Relat Res 2016;474(9):1957–61.
15. Association of American Medical Colleges. Table 1.3. Number and Percentage of Active Physicians by Sex and Specialty.; 2017. Available at: https://www.aamc.

org/data-reports/workforce/interactive-data/active-physicians-sex-and-specialty-2017. Accessed October 1, 2022.
16. Belk JW, Littlefield CP, Mulcahey MK, et al. Characteristics of Orthopaedic Sports Medicine Fellowship Directors. Orthop J Sports Med 2021;9(2):2325967120985257.
17. Kamalapathy P, Moore A, Brockmeier S, et al. Status Quo: Trends in Diversity and Unique Traits Among Orthopaedic Sports Medicine Fellowship Directors. J Am Acad Orthop Surg 2022;30(1):36–43.
18. Schiller NC, Sama AJ, Spielman AF, et al. Trends in leadership at orthopaedic surgery sports medicine fellowships. World J Orthop 2021;12(6):412–22.
19. Shah KN, Ruddell JH, Scott B, et al. Orthopaedic Surgery Faculty: An Evaluation of Gender and Racial Diversity Compared with Other Specialties. JB JS Open Access 2020;5(3):e2000009.
20. Maqsoodi N, Mesfin A, Li X. Academic, Leadership, and Demographic Characteristics of Orthopaedic Sports Medicine Division Chiefs in the United States. J Am Acad Orthop Surg Glob Res Rev 2022;6(1). https://doi.org/10.5435/JAAOSGlobal-D-21-00139.
21. Peck CJ, Schmidt SJ, Latimore DA, et al. Chair Versus Chairman: Does Orthopaedics Use the Gendered Term More Than Other Specialties? Clin Orthop Relat Res 2020;478(7):1583–9.
22. O'Reilly OC, Day MA, Cates WT, et al. Female Team Physician Representation in Professional and Collegiate Athletics. Am J Sports Med 2020;48(3):739–43.
23. Hinkle AJ, Brown SM, Mulcahey MK. Gender disparity among NBA and WNBA team physicians. Phys Sportsmed 2021;49(2):219–22.
24. Wiggins AJ, Agha O, Diaz A, et al. Current Perceptions of Diversity Among Head Team Physicians and Head Athletic Trainers: Results Across US Professional Sports Leagues. Orthop J Sports Med 2021;9(10):23259671211047270.
25. Kim CY, Sivasundaram L, Trivedi NN, et al. A 46-year Analysis of Gender Trends in Academic Authorship in Orthopaedic Sports Medicine. J Am Acad Orthop Surg 2019;27(13):493–501.
26. Rynecki ND, Krell ES, Potter JS, et al. How Well Represented Are Women Orthopaedic Surgeons and Residents on Major Orthopaedic Editorial Boards and Publications? Clin Orthop Relat Res 2020;478(7):1563–8.
27. Hiller KP, Boulos A, Tran MM, et al. What Are the Rates and Trends of Women Authors in Three High-impact Orthopaedic Journals from 2006-2017? Clin Orthop Relat Res 2020;478(7):1553–60.
28. Brown MA, Erdman MK, Munger AM, et al. Despite Growing Number of Women Surgeons, Authorship Gender Disparity in Orthopaedic Literature Persists Over 30 Years. Clin Orthop Relat Res 2020;478(7):1542–52.
29. Potter JS, Ranpura A, Rynecki ND, et al. Gender Parity in Academic Leadership Roles at AOSSM Annual Meetings. Orthop J Sports Med 2021;9(1):2325967120979995.
30. Gerull KM, Kim DJ, Cogsil T, et al. Are Women Proportionately Represented as Speakers at Orthopaedic Surgery Annual Meetings? A Cross-Sectional Analysis. Clin Orthop Relat Res 2020;478(12):2729–40.
31. National Federation of State High School Associations. 2017-2018 High School Athletics Participation Survey.; 2018. https://www.nfhs.org/media/1020205/2017-18_hs_participation_survey.pdf. Accessed October 1, 2022.
32. Bassett AJ, Ahlmen A, Rosendorf JM, et al. The Biology of Sex and Sport. JBJS Rev 2020;8(3):e0140.

33. Carter CW, Ireland ML, Johnson AE, et al. Sex-based Differences in Common Sports Injuries. J Am Acad Orthop Surg 2018;26(13):447–54.
34. Flaxman TE, Smith AJJ, Benoit DL. Sex-related differences in neuromuscular control: Implications for injury mechanisms or healthy stabilisation strategies? J Orthop Res 2014;32(2):310–7.
35. Wolf JM, Cannada L, Van Heest AE, et al. Male and female differences in musculoskeletal disease. J Am Acad Orthop Surg 2015;23(6):339–47.
36. Hilibrand MJ, Hammoud S, Bishop M, et al. Common injuries and ailments of the female athlete; pathophysiology, treatment and prevention. Phys Sportsmed 2015;43(4):403–11.
37. Marar M, McIlvain NM, Fields SK, et al. Epidemiology of concussions among United States high school athletes in 20 sports. Am J Sports Med 2012;40(4): 747–55.
38. Covassin T, Elbin RJ, Harris W, et al. The role of age and sex in symptoms, neurocognitive performance, and postural stability in athletes after concussion. Am J Sports Med 2012;40(6):1303–12.
39. Doherty C, Delahunt E, Caulfield B, et al. The incidence and prevalence of ankle sprain injury: a systematic review and meta-analysis of prospective epidemiological studies. Sports Med 2014;44(1):123–40.
40. Merrill A, Guzman K, Miller SL. Gender differences in glenoid anatomy: an anatomic study. Surg Radiol Anat 2009;31(3):183–9.
41. Hayes MK, Brown S, Mulcahey MK. Women's Sports Medicine Programs in the United States: an interdisciplinary approach to the care of girls and women. Phys Sportsmed 2020;48(1):81–5.
42. Tanaka MJ, Szymanski LM, Dale JL, et al. Team Approach: Treatment of Injuries in the Female Athlete: Multidisciplinary Considerations for Women's Sports Medicine Programs. JBJS Rev 2019;7(1):e7.
43. Nielsen MW, Andersen JP, Schiebinger L, et al. One and a half million medical papers reveal a link between author gender and attention to gender and sex analysis. Nat Hum Behav 2017;1(11):791–6.
44. Sugimoto CR, Ahn YY, Smith E, et al. Factors affecting sex-related reporting in medical research: a cross-disciplinary bibliometric analysis. Lancet 2019; 393(10171):550–9.
45. Baldwin K, Namdari S, Bowers A, et al. Factors affecting interest in orthopedics among female medical students: a prospective analysis. Orthopedics 2011; 34(12):e919–32.
46. Hill JF, Yule A, Zurakowski D, et al. Residents' perceptions of sex diversity in orthopaedic surgery. J Bone Joint Surg Am 2013;95(19):e1441–6.
47. O'Connor MI. Medical School Experiences Shape Women Students' Interest in Orthopaedic Surgery. Clin Orthop Relat Res 2016;474(9):1967–72.
48. Bernstein J, Dicaprio MR, Mehta S. The relationship between required medical school instruction in musculoskeletal medicine and application rates to orthopaedic surgery residency programs. J Bone Joint Surg Am 2004;86(10):2335–8.
49. Rahman R, Zhang B, Humbyrd CJ, et al. How Do Medical Students Perceive Diversity in Orthopaedic Surgery, and How Do Their Perceptions Change After an Orthopaedic Clinical Rotation? Clin Orthop Relat Res 2021;479(3):434–44.
50. Johnson AL, Sharma J, Chinchilli VM, et al. Why do medical students choose orthopaedics as a career? J Bone Joint Surg Am 2012;94(11):e78.
51. Weiss J, Caird MS. Editorial Comment: Women and Underrepresented Minorities in Orthopaedics. Clin Orthop Relat Res 2016;474(9):1943–4.

52. Harbold D, Dearolf L, Buckley J, et al. The Perry Initiative's Impact on Gender Diversity Within Orthopedic Education. Curr Rev Musculoskelet Med 2021;14(6):429–33.
53. Coffin MD, Collins CS, Dib AG, et al. A Plausible Pipeline to Diversifying Orthopaedics: Premedical Programming. J Surg Educ 2022;79(1):122–8.
54. Lattanza LL, Meszaros-Dearolf L, O'Connor MI, et al. The Perry Initiative's Medical Student Outreach Program Recruits Women Into Orthopaedic Residency. Clin Orthop Relat Res 2016;474(9):1962–6.
55. Mason BS, Ross W, Ortega G, et al. Can a Strategic Pipeline Initiative Increase the Number of Women and Underrepresented Minorities in Orthopaedic Surgery? Clin Orthop Relat Res 2016;474(9):1979–85.
56. Jagsi R, Griffith KA, DeCastro RA, et al. Sex, role models, and specialty choices among graduates of US medical schools in 2006-2008. J Am Coll Surg 2014; 218(3):345–52.
57. Okike K, Phillips DP, Swart E, et al. Orthopaedic Faculty and Resident Sex Diversity Are Associated with the Orthopaedic Residency Application Rate of Female Medical Students. J Bone Joint Surg Am 2019;101(12):e56.
58. Cannada LK, O'Connor MI. Equity360: Gender, Race, and Ethnicity-Harassment in Orthopaedics and #SpeakUpOrtho. Clin Orthop Relat Res 2021;479(8):1674–6.
59. Robin JX, Murali S, Paul KD, et al. Disparities Among Industry's Highly Compensated Orthopaedic Surgeons. JB JS Open Access 2021;6(4):e21.
60. Buerba RA, Arshi A, Greenberg DC, et al. The Role of Gender, Academic Affiliation, and Subspecialty in Relation to Industry Payments to Orthopaedic Surgeons. J Natl Med Assoc 2020;112(1):82–90.
61. Poon S, Luong M, Hargett D, et al. Does a Career in Orthopaedic Surgery Affect a Woman's Fertility? J Am Acad Orthop Surg 2021;29(5):e243–50.
62. Hamilton AR, Tyson MD, Braga JA, et al. Childbearing and pregnancy characteristics of female orthopaedic surgeons. J Bone Joint Surg Am 2012;94(11):e77.
63. Reid DBC, Shah KN, Lama CJ, et al. Parenthood Among Orthopedic Surgery Residents: Assessment of Resident and Program Director Perceptions on Training. Orthopedics 2021;44(2):98–104.
64. Nemeth C, Roll E, Mulcahey MK. Program Directors' Perception of Pregnancy and Parenthood in Orthopedic Surgery Residency. Orthopedics 2020;43(2):e109–13.
65. Clement RC, Olsson E, Katti P, et al. Fringe Benefits Among US Orthopedic Residency Programs Vary Considerably: a National Survey. HSS J 2016;12(2):158–64.
66. Compton J, Hajewski CJ, Pugely AJ. Pregnancy and Parental Leave During Orthopaedic Surgery Residency. Iowa Orthop J 2021;41(1):19–23.
67. Hern HG, Trivedi T, Alter HJ, et al. How Prevalent Are Potentially Illegal Questions During Residency Interviews? A Follow-up Study of Applicants to All Specialties in the National Resident Matching Program. Acad Med 2016;91(11):1546–53.
68. Huntington WP, Haines N, Patt JC. What factors influence applicants' rankings of orthopaedic surgery residency programs in the National Resident Matching Program? Clin Orthop Relat Res 2014;472(9):2859–66.
69. Balch Samora J, Van Heest A, Weber K, et al. Discrimination, and Bullying in Orthopaedics: A Work Environment and Culture Survey. J Am Acad Orthop Surg 2020;28(24):e1097–104.
70. Whicker E, Williams C, Kirchner G, et al. What Proportion of Women Orthopaedic Surgeons Report Having Been Sexually Harassed During Residency Training? A Survey Study. Clin Orthop Relat Res 2020;478(11):2598–606.
71. Gianakos AL, Mulcahey MK, Weiss JM, et al. #SpeakUpOrtho: Narratives of Women in Orthopaedic Surgery-Invited Manuscript. J Am Acad Orthop Surg 2022;30(8):369–76.

Racial and Ethnic Disparities in Sports Medicine and the Importance of Diversity

Kellie K. Middleton, MD, MPH[a,*], Alex Turner, BS, BA[b]

KEYWORDS

• Diversity • Healthcare disparities • Head team physicians • Sports medicine
• Orthopedic surgery • Minority athletes • Race • Underrepresented minority (URM)

KEY POINTS

- According to the Association of American Medical Colleges, the racial and ethnic composition of the country's physician work force does not reflect that of the general population.
- Within orthopedic surgery, the absence of underrepresented minorities is greatest for the subspecializations of sports medicine, spine, and trauma.
- Black/African American and Latino/Hispanic head team physicians are significantly underrepresented when it comes to the health care of a diverse athlete population.
- Within the sports medicine specialty, there are significant differences in access to care and time to definitive treatment between White patients and patients of color.
- Increased diversity is correlated with improvements in physician–patient relationship (affecting communication and decision making) and patient satisfaction.

INTRODUCTION

The United States is becoming more diverse with each passing census. The 2020 US Census bureau revealed that 57.8% of the population was White alone (not Hispanic or Latino), a decrease from 63.7% in 2010. The second largest racial/ethnic group in 2020 was Hispanic or Latino making up 18.7% of the population (increased from 16.3% in 2010). The third largest racial/ethnic group was Black or African American alone (not Hispanic or Latino), which comprised 12.1% and 12.2% of the US population in 2020 and 2010, respectively.[1] Asian Americans currently make up 5.9% of the US population, Native Americans or Alaska Natives make up 0.7%, and individuals who identify as 2 or more races comprise 4.1%. The increasing percentages of minority populations has impacted the way americans view their individuality. The once coined "melting pot" of America is now more accurately described as a "salad bowl" in which *diversity* is celebrated along with oneness.

[a] Northside Hospital, Atlanta, GA, USA; [b] University of Texas Southwestern Medical School, Dallas, TX, USA
* Corresponding author. 771 Old Norcross Road, suite 105, Lawrenceville, GA 30046.
E-mail address: kelmd6@gmail.com

Clin Sports Med 43 (2024) 233–244
https://doi.org/10.1016/j.csm.2023.07.005
0278-5919/24/

The changing face of our country as a whole is also being emulated at the community level, as diversity increases within various independent fields. Commercial industry, educational institutions, and health care systems embrace the clear advantages and economic benefits of diversity.[2–4] For instance, Deloitte employees self-reported that their organization is better able to innovate, is more responsive to changing customer needs, and is overall better at team collaborating when the organization committed to and supported diversity.[5] Deloitte found that both inclusion and diversity were important to overall team success.

Nonetheless, some fields demographically fail to parallel the increasing diversity of the United States. According to the Association of American Medical Colleges (AAMC), the racial and ethnic composition of the country's physician work force does not reflect that of the general population.[6] This contributes to health care disparities with regard to access, administration of care, and patient outcomes.[7,8] Some medical specialties fare better than others in terms of ethnic and racial diversity. H One of the least diverse specialties is that of orthopedic surgery. As a surgical subspecialty, orthopedics has the lowest representation of minorities, with a significant decrease in diversity over an 11 year period.[9] Within orthopedic subspecialties, sports medicine is the least diverse. The lack of diversity in orthopedic sports medicine may demonstrate one of the greatest discrepancies in minority representation between the athlete patient and provider populations.

In this paper, we will discuss the benefits of diversity and its implications in health care, specifically within orthopedic surgery and its subspecialty of sports medicine. We will provide recommendations for improving diversity in sports medicine to better serve the racially and ethnically diverse athletic populations.

ORTHOPEDIC SURGERY DIVERSITY (OR LACK THEREOF)

Racial and ethnic groups whose representation in socioeconomics, education, and employment is smaller than their representation in the US population are defined as underrepresented minority (URM) groups.[10,11] By this definition, the AAMC specifies Blacks or African Americans, Hispanics or Latinos, and American Indians or Alaskan Natives as URM groups within the physician workforce and the population of students graduating from medical school.[12]

Data from the US Census Bureau, the Accreditation Council for Graduate Medical Education (ACGME), and the American Academy of Orthopedic Surgeons (AAOS) reveal that orthopedic surgery is the least diverse of all surgical subspecialties.[13] Although the number of URM in orthopedic surgery has increased over the last 2 decades, it is doing so at a slower rate compared with other surgical and nonsurgical subspecialties.[14–17] This makes the orthopedic surgery specialty one of the least representative of the racial and ethnic composition of the United States.

Within orthopedic surgery, the absence of URMs is greatest for the subspecializations of sports medicine, spine, and trauma.[18] According to Poon and colleagues,[18] sports medicine recruited a significantly greater percentage of white fellows compared with musculoskeletal oncology, pediatrics, adult reconstruction, and spine. Furthermore, Maqsoodi and colleagues[19] found that the number of fellowship programs without a single URM rose from 40 programs in 2002 to 60 programs in 2016 (reaching a high of 76 programs in 2011). In contrast, of the 82 fellowship programs, the number of programs per year with more than one URM fell from 61 programs in 2002 to 53 programs in 2016. In 2010, this number was as low as 31.

When evaluating the orthopedic pipeline, racial/ethnic diversity is lacking in residency programs,[9] fellowship programs,[18] and orthopedic faculty.[20,21] Poon and colleagues found that between 2006 and 2015, there was no change in ethnic diversity among orthopedic fellows, indicating that there had been no significant change within orthopedic surgery subspecialties. A lack of diversity at leadership levels clearly influences the disparities observed in residency and fellowship programs. Nearly 98% of the sports medicine fellowship directors (FDs) were male and 84% were White.[22] Of the 16% belonging to racial/ethnic groups, 7.32% were Asian Americans, 2.44% Hispanic/Latino, 2.44% African American, and 3.66% were of another race/ethnicity.

Schiller and colleagues[22] revealed that 69.5% of current sports medicine FDs served as team physicians for US professional baseball, football, hockey, basketball, and soccer teams. FDs are more likely to become team physicians for university-wide athletics and provide care for all affiliated sports teams. Thus, being in a leadership position such as FD creates greater opportunities for sports medicine physicians to hold appointments as a team physician and to directly impact the care of collegiate and professional athletes. This is significant with regard to health disparities considering a large majority of collegiate and professional athletes in football, basketball, and track & field are URMs.

Racial/Ethnic Diversity in High-Level Sports

Collegiate athletes

The National Collegiate Athletics Association (NCAA) Demographics Database includes self-reported data from active NCAA programs between 2011 and 2022.[23] Gender, race, and ethnicity information was reported for athletes and administrative and coaching positions within the athletic department including full- and part-time coaching staff as well as volunteers. Including Historically Black Colleges and Universities (HBCUs), 35% of 2022 Division-I student-athletes were a person of color (POC).

POC includes those who are non-White but excludes those who identified as "international" or whose race was "unknown." As a result, the percent of POC may be underestimated.

The top 3 Division I men's sports with the greatest number of persons of color (POCs) were basketball (estimated 77% POC), football (estimated 64% POC), and soccer (estimated 55%). For Division I women's sports, basketball (estimated 69% POC), indoor and outdoor track and field (estimated 47% POC), gymnastics (estimated 39% POC), and soccer (estimated 36% POC), were the top sports with the greatest diversity.[24]

The Racial and Gender Report Card (RGRC), issued by The Institute for Diversity and Ethics in Sport (TIDES), provides an assessment of racial/ethnic and gender hiring practices in most of the leading professional and amateur sports and sporting organizations in the United States.[25] The primary goal of publishing the RGRC is to promote diversity within athletic departments and ensure equity in hiring practices, particularly given the percentage of URM athletes in high revenue sports.

Professional sports

Of all professional sports RGRCs, the Women's National Basketball Association (WNBA) scored the highest. In the 2021 WNBA season, 19.9% of the players were White whereas 74.5% of players were Black/African American, 3.5% of players identified as 2 or more races. That is, 80.1% of WNBA athletes identify as "persons of color" (POC). With the best representation of POCs, the WNBA earned an "A+" overall on the RGRC, an "A+" for racial hiring. The only men's leagues close to comparison with regard to diversity hiring and representation of POC were the National Basketball Association (NBA) and Major League Soccer (MLS).

The NBA received an "A" grade overall with an "A+" in racial hiring for the 2022 RGRC. Only 17.4% of the NBA players are White; 82.4% of players are POC: 71.8% of players were Black/African American, 8% were categorized as "two or more races/ other", 2.4% of players were Hispanic/Latino, and 0.2% were Asian. Half of the coaches and assistant coaches in the NBA are POC with 46.7% of the coaches and 42.7% of the assistant coaches, respectively, identifying as Black/African American.[26]

MLS earned an overall grade of "B" for the 2021 RGRC, but an "A+" grade for player diversity. Of the 61.7% POC comprising the MLS rosters, 31.6% of players were Hispanic/Latino, 24.1% Black/African Americans, 1.3% Asian, 0.2% Hawaiian/Pacific Islander, 0.4% American Indian/Alaskan Native, and 4% identified as being 2 or more races.[27]

The National Football League (NFL) received an "A+" for diversity within the player population, but "B" overall and a "B+" for racial hiring according to the 2021 RGRC. Similar to the NBA, 70.7% of the league is composed of POCs with 58% of players identifying as Black/African American and 9.8% of players identifying as 2 or more races. One-quarter of NFL players are White, 1.6% are Native Hawaiians or Pacific Islanders, 0.7% are Hispanic/Latino, 0.2% Alaska Native or American Indian, and 0.1% Asian. A little over 4% of NFL players chose not to specify their race.[28]

Major League Baseball (MLB) earned an "A+" in player demographics with 38% of players being POC (28.5% Hispanic/Latino, 7.2% Black/African American, 1.9% Asian, 0.3% Hawaiian/Pacific Islanders, and 0.1% Native American). Additionally, 275 (28.2%) players represent 21 different countries and territories outside of the 50 United States in 2022. Sixty-two percent of MLB players and 80% of MLB managers are White.[29]

Interestingly, diversity within the head athletic training staff was included in the RGRC for the NBA, WNBA, and MLS; however, demographics of head team physicians (HTPs) were not analyzed.

Head team physicians

Neither the NCAA Demographics Database nor the RGRC collect racial/ethnic demographic data on medical staff including team physicians (orthopedic surgeons and primary care specialists). However, a recent study by Wiggins and colleagues[30] evaluated the level of diversity of HTP and head athletic trainers (ATCs) within men's professional sports leagues in the United States. The majority of professional team HTPs were orthopedic surgeons (78%); however, alternate specialties included primary care sports medicine, family medicine or physical medicine, and rehabilitation. Two observers analyzed photographs and names of medical staff to determine his or her perceived race and sex with disagreements resolved by a third independent observer. They found that within the NBA, NFL, MLS and MLB, only 15.5% of HTPs were POC: 8.4% were classified as Asian, 5.8% Black, 1.3% Hispanic/Latino, 0% Native American.[30]

There is limited data with respect to HTPs in female professional sports. Wilson and colleagues found that 20.8% of HTPs in the WNBA, National Women's Soccer League, and National Women's Hockey League were minority.[31] Three of 24 (the largest proportion of the minority cohort) HTPs were Black. The WNBA had the highest percentage of perceived minority HTPs at 30%, all of whom were Black. Compared to men's professional leagues, 54.2% of women's professional leagues HTPs were orthopedic surgeons. Other specialties included family medicine, physical medication and rehabilitation, and pediatrics.

For perspective, 17.4% of NBA athletes are White and 76.7% of HTPs are White. Similarly in the NFL, 25% of the athletes are White and 88.2% of HTPs are White.

For MLS and MLB, 31.6% and 28.5% of the athletes, respectively, identified as Latino/Hispanic according to the RGRC results. However, there are no Latino/Hispanic HTPs in either professional league with 84.6% and 86.7% of the HTPs being White in MLS and MLB, respectively. In the WNBA, 80.1% of the players and 30% of HTPs are POC (**Fig. 1**).

Above are just a few examples of the demographic discrepancies between health care providers and the athletes that they serve. Black/African American and Latino/Hispanic HTPs are significantly underrepresented when it comes to the health care of a diverse athlete population.

Racial and Ethnic Disparities in Orthopedics

Racial and ethnic disparities in health care access and quality have been extensively documented. Research has shown that racial/ethnic minorities have less access to care even after controlling for income,[32–34] and that they have worse medical outcomes in various fields including adult reconstruction and spine surgery.[35,36] Black and Hispanic patients with calcaneus fractures were less likely to undergo open reduction and internal fixation as compared to White patients.[37] Similarly, higher rates of fixation of clavicle fractures were found in patients who were White, were privately insured, and were of a higher socioeconomic status.[38]

Although there have been no major significant differences in outcomes following sports-related surgeries, there are significant differences in access to care and time to definitive treatment between White patients and patients of color. Two of the most common sports-related knee injuries are anterior cruciate ligament (ACL) tears and meniscus tears. White patients are more likely than non-White patients to undergo ACL reconstruction after an ACL injury is diagnosed.[39] In pediatric and adolescent populations, Black and Hispanic patients experienced greater surgical delays after ACL tear.[40] Additionally, Black and Hispanic children have more irreparable meniscus tears (influenced by surgical delay) and less physical therapy visits likely contributing

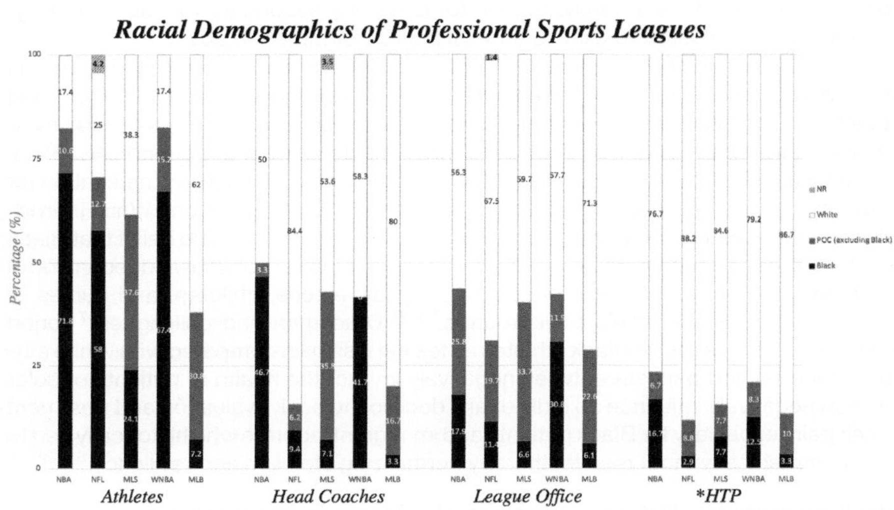

Fig. 1. Head team physicians (HTP) statistics based on Wiggins and colleagues (all sports excluding the WNBA) and Wilson and colleagues (WNBA) demonstrating disparity between athlete-patients and head team physicians (HTP). * defines HTP as head team physicians and also cites from where the numbers were extracted (2 different cites).

to the finding of greater residual hamstring and quadriceps weakness 9 months postoperatively.[40]

With respect to rotator cuff repair, another common orthopedic sports procedure, Black race, Hispanic/Latino ethnicity, and government insurance (eg, Medicaid) were independently associated with lower rates of operative management.[41] In shoulder arthroplasty, the disparity gaps continue to be sizable with Black patients having a higher rate of nonhome discharge, longer length of stay, and higher costs associated with surgery. Hispanic patients also have a longer length of stay and higher costs compared with White patients.[42]

Outside of musculoskeletal sports-related injuries, head injuries are also a common occurrence highlighting racial differences in diagnosis, treatment, and education on sports-related concussion (SRC). Wallace and colleagues[43] found that Black adolescent athletes exhibited less knowledge regarding concussion and were less likely to recognize symptoms compared to their White counterparts. Without timely and accurate diagnosis, athletes may prematurely return to play, potentially exacerbating mild traumatic brain injury and increasing the risk for second-impact syndrome.[44,45] Black patients were less likely to have emergency department (ED) visits for head injuries or concussions and were less likely to be diagnosed with a concussion during an ED visit.[46] Moreover, Black athletes have a greater risk of neurocognitive impairment following SRC.[47] Race and ethnicity were also associated with reporting a suicide attempt after experiencing an SRC. American Indians or Alaska Natives were the racial/ethnicity groups with the highest risks of suicide attempt (odds ration [OR] 2.00; 95% confidence interval [CI], 1.37–2.91), followed by multiracial (OR 1.66; 95% CI, 1.38–2.01), Black (OR, 1.21; 95% CI, 1.06–1.37), and Hispanic/Latino (OR 1.21; 95% CI; 1.07–1.36) compared with youth who identified as White.[48]

In the 1990s, the NFL used race as a determining factor affecting the NFL's $1 billion concussion settlement for former NFL athletes with dementia. "Race-norming" assumed Black players started out with lower cognitive function, and thus, deserved less than White players.[49,50] After months of legal negotiations, Black retired football players who were denied compensation for dementia secondary to "race-norming" can now be re-evaluated to eliminate racial bias as of March 4, 2021.[51]

Not only has prejudicial perceived cognitive performance and intelligence based on race harmed athletes of color, health care providers preconceived notions regarding patient pain has also negatively impacted the care of Black patients.[52] In a study evaluating the allocation of pain medication in children diagnosed with appendicitis, Black children were significantly less likely than White children to receive any medication for moderate pain and were less likely to receive opioids.[53] Both Black and White individuals have race-related stereotypes concerning pain perception.[54] The belief that Black people feel less pain than White people has been extensively acknowledged in social psychology literature with false beliefs held by laypersons, children, and nurses of both White and Black ethnic backgrounds.[55,56] Druckman and colleagues[57] found that medical staff perceive Black athletes as feeling less pain compared with White athletes. Race-related pain stereotypes negatively impact the health of patients of color and also negatively influence an individual's decision to seek evaluation and treatment of their pain, especially for Black patients and immigrant laborers who historically had to endure hardships without respite, thereby normalizing stoicism and resiliency.[58–62]

Why Representation Matters: Importance of Diversity in Sports Medicine

In 2016, 305 members of the American Orthopedic Association (AOA) completed a survey evaluating their knowledge of racial/ethnic disparities and their perceptions on the underlying causes.[63] The majority of respondents were White and male (78%

and 88%, respectively). Nearly half (46%) of the respondents reported caring for patient populations in which one-fourth or less of the patients were minorities. Sixty-eight percent of the respondents acknowledge that there is at least some evidence of disparities in orthopedic care; however, the majority attributed this to health insurance (or a lack thereof) and a higher burden of comorbidities. More than half (58%) of the respondents felt that racial/ethnic differences "never" exist in their own practices. The authors concluded that although 83% of the respondents believe that racial/ethnic disparities in orthopedics are important to address, "self-awareness" is lacking among AOA orthopedic surgeons and residents as a group.

At a group level, people tend to favor in-group members over outgroups, even when in-group similarities are nonexistent.[64] In this environment, individuals tend to approach outgroups with uncertainty and vigilance, potentially resulting in negative attitudes.[65] Such attitudes are more likely to occur in a homogenous setting. At an individual level, people show homophily, or demonstrating attraction to others perceived as similar.[66] One would believe this to be related to race; however, Byrne and Wong in 1962 found that similarities can transcend race and/or may not be related to an individual's preference.[67]

Increased diversity is correlated with improvements in physician–patient relationship (affecting communication and decision making) and patient satisfaction. Gomez and colleagues[4] demonstrated that patient outcomes are better when care is provided by a more diverse team. Furthermore, perceived personal similarity and patient–physician racial concordance led to higher ratings of trust, patient satisfaction, and intention to adhere to physician recommendations.[68] Patients in race-concordant relationships with their physicians also experience greater participation and satisfaction during health visits and have longer visit times.[69–72] Of note, some may argue that homophily is occurring when patients prefer same-gender or same-race physicians; however, this is not the case. There are many other factors to consider particularly given the established racial disparities in medicine. Additionally, Black patients may prefer race-concordant physicians in the setting of known racial biases in society, medical distrust arising from historical experimentation, exploitation, and continued racial health care disparities in America outside the scope of this article.[73–75] Additionally, race concordance can increase the probability that the patient and clinician speak the same language, though this may not always be the case. Lastly, White patients are the most likely to have a same race clinician (46%), significantly more compared with Black, Latino, or Asian patients.[76]

Conceivably, diversity and inclusion will help decrease stereotype dispersion, and in turn, bias.[77] Diverse environments are more likely to expose individuals to variation, thus encountering "stereotype-(in)consistent" experiences that challenge prior held stereotypes.[78,79] Bai and colleagues found that this correlates positively with subjective wellbeing. Hence, why efforts should be made particularly in health care to create a diverse physician workforce better serve diverse patient populations. Given the longstanding role of orthopedic surgeons in the care of collegiate and professional athletes, the demographics of the medical staff are an important component to consider in the care of diverse athlete patient populations within universities and professional franchises in the United States.

CLINICS CARE POINTS

- When evaluating the orthopaedic pipeline, racial/ethnic diversity is lacking in residency programs,[20] fellowship programs[21] and orthopaedic faculty.[22,23]

- Nearly 98% of the sports medicine fellowship directors (FDs) were male and 84% were White.[24]
- Over sixty-nine% of current sports medicine FDs served as team physicians for US professional baseball, football, hockey, basketball, and soccer teams. FDs are more likely to become team physicians for university-wide athletics and provide care for all affiliated sports teams.
- A large majority of collegiate and professional athletes in football, men's and women's basketball, and men's and women's track & field are underrepresented minorities (URMs).
- The top three Division I men's sports with the greatest number of persons of color (POCs) were basketball (estimated 77% POC), football (estimated 64% POC), and soccer (estimated 55%).
- For Division I women's sports, basketball (estimated 69% POC), indoor and outdoor track and field (estimated 47% POC), gymnastics (estimated 39% POC), and soccer (estimated 36% POC), were the top sports with the greatest diversity.[26]
- Within the NBA, NFL, MLS and MLB, only 15.5% of head team physicians (HTPs) were POC: 8.4% were classified as Asian, 5.8% Black, 1.3% Hispanic/Latino, 0% Native American.[33]
- Patients in race-concordant relationships with their physicians experience greater participation and satisfaction during office health visits and have longer visit times.[74,75,76,77]

DISCLOSURE

The authors declare that they have no relevant or material financial interests that relate to the research described in this article.

REFERENCES

1. United States Census Bureau. 2020. Available at: https://www.census.gov/library/visualizations/interactive/racial-and-ethnic-diversity-in-the-united-states-2010-and-2020-census.html. https://www.census.gov/library/stories/2021/08/2020-united-states-population-more-racially-ethnically-diverse-than-2010.html.
2. Cook A, Glass C. Diversity begets diversity? The effects of board composition on the appointment and success of women CEOs. Soc Sci Res 2015;53:137–47.
3. Elliott JR, Smith RA. Ethnic matching of supervisors to subordinate work groups: Findings on "bottom-up" ascription and social closure. Soc Probl 2001;48(2): 258–76.
4. Gomez LE, Bernet P. Diversity improves performance and outcomes. J of the National Medical Association 2019;111(4):383–92.
5. Bourke J, Dillon B. Waiter is that inclusion in my soup? A new recipe to improve business performance. Deloitte and the Victorian Equal Opportunity and Human Rights Commission, 2013, Sydney, Australia.
6. HIS Markit Ltd. The complexities of physicians supply and demand: projections from 2018 to 2034. Washington, DC: AAMC; 2021.
7. Jackson CS, Gracia JN. Addressing health and healtht-care disparities: the role of a diverse work-force and the social determinants of health. Publ Health Rep 2014;129(2):57–61.
8. Rivo ML, Satcher D. Improving access to healthcare through physician workforce reform: directions for the 21st century. JAMA 1993;270(9):1074–8.
9. Poon S, Kiridly D, Mutawakkil M, et al. Current Trends in Sex, Race, and Ethnic Diversity in Orthopaedic Surgery Residency. J Am Acad Orthop Surg 2019; 27(16):e725–33.

10. Bhatti HA. Toward "Inclusifying" the underrepresented minority in STEM education research. J Microbiol Biol Educ 2021;22(3):e211.
11. Page KR, Castillo-Page L, Poll-Hunter N, et al. Assessing the evolving definition of underrepresented minority and its application in. academic medicine. Acad Med. 2013;88(1):67–72.
12. Templeton K, Wood VJ, Haynes R. Women and minorities in orthopaedic residency programs. JAAOS 2007;15(1):S37–41.
13. Ramirez RN, Franklin CC. Racial diversity in orthopaedic surgery. Orthop Clin North Am 2019;50:337–44.
14. Shah KN, Ruddell JH, Scott B, et al. Orthopaedic Surgery Faculty: An Evaluation of Gender and Racial Diversity Compared with Other Specialties. JB JS. Open Access 2020;5(3):e20.00009.
15. Jarman BT, Borgert AJ, Kallies KJ, et al. Underrepresented Minorities in General Surgery Residency: Analysis of Interviewed Applicants, Residents, and Core Teaching Faculty. J Am Coll Surg 2020;231(1):54–8.
16. McDonald TC, Drake LC, Replogle WH, et al. Barriers to Increasing Diversity in Orthopaedics: The Residency Program Perspective. JB JS. Open Access 2020;5(2):e0007.
17. England SP, Pierce RO Jr. Current diversity in orthopaedics. Issues of race, ethnicity, and gender. CORR 1999;362:40–3.
18. Poon S, Kiridly D, Brown L, et al. Evaluation of Sex, Ethnic, and Racial Diversity Across US ACGME-Accredited Orthopedic Subspecialty Fellowship Programs. Orthopedics 2018;41(5):282–8.
19. Maqsoodi N, Mesfinn A, Li X. Academic, leadership, and demographic characteristics of orthopaedic sports medicine division chiefs in the United States. JAAOS Global Research & Reviews 2022;6(1):1–6.
20. Chen RE, Kuhns BD, Kaupp S, et al. Diversity among academic orthopedic shoulder and elbow surgery faculty in the United States. J Shoulder Elbow Surg 2020;29(4):655–9.
21. Day CS, Lage DE, Ahn CS. Diversity based on race, ethnicity, and sex between academic orthopaedic surgery and other specialties: a comparative study. J Bone Joint Surg Am 2010;92(13):2328–35.
22. Schiller NC, Sama AJ, Spielman AF, et al. Trends in leadership at orthopaedic surgery sports medicine fellowships. World J Orthop 2021;12(6):412–22.
23. NCAA Demographics Database. Available at: https://www.ncaa.org/sports/2018/12/13/ncaa-demographics-database.aspx. Accessed Nov. 5, 2022.
24. NCAA Demographics Database. Available at: https://www.ncaa.org/sports/2018/12/13/ncaa-demographics-database.aspx. Accessed May 27, 2023.
25. Lapchick RE. The 2021 racial and gender Report card: College sports. The Institute for diversity and Ethics in sport (TIDES). Orlando, FL: University of Central Florida; 2021.
26. Lapchick RE. The 2022 racial and gender Report card: National basketball Association. The Institute for diversity and Ethics in sport (TIDES). Orlando, FL: University of Central Florida; 2022.
27. Lapchick RE. The 2021 racial and gender Report card: major league soccer. The Institute for diversity and Ethics in sport (TIDES). Orlando, FL: University of Central Florida; 2021.
28. Lapchick RE. The 2021 racial and gender Report card: National football league. The Institute for diversity and Ethics in sport (TIDES). Orlando, FL: University of Central Florida; 2021.

29. Lapchick RE. The 2022 racial and gender Report card: major league baseball. The Institute for diversity and Ethics in sport (TIDES). Orlando, FL: University of Central Florida; 2022.
30. Wiggins AJ, Agha O, Diaz A, et al. Current Perceptions of Diversity Among Head Team Physicians and Head Athletic Trainers: Results Across US Professional Sports Leagues. Orthop J Sports Med 2021;9(10). 23259671211047271.
31. Wilson J, Agha O, Wiggins AJ, et al. Gender and Racial Diversity Among the Head Medical and Athletic Training Staff of Women's Professional Sports Leagues. Orthop J Sports Med 2023;11(2). 23259671221150447.
32. Jancuska JM, Hutzler L, Protopsaltis TS, et al. Utilization of Lumbar Spinal Fusion in New York State: Trends and Disparities. Spine 2016;41(19):1508–14.
33. Singgh JA, Ramachandran R. Persisting racial disparities in total shoulder arthroplasty (TSA) utilization and outcomes. Journal of Racial and Ethnic Health Disparities 2016;3:259–66.
34. Yu S, Mahure SA, Branch N, et al. Impact of Race and Gender on Utilization Rate of Total Shoulder Arthroplasty. Orthopedics 2016;39(3):e538–44.
35. Schoenfeld AJ, Tipirneni R, Nelson JH, et al. The influence of race and ethnicity on complications and mortality after orthopaedic surgery. Med Care 2014;52: 842–51.
36. Ibrahim SA, Stone RA, Han X, et al. Racial/ethnic differences in surgical outcomes in veterans following knee or hip arthroplasty. Arthritis Rheum 2005; 52(10):3143–51.
37. Zelle BA, Morton-Gonzaba NA, Adcock CF, et al. Healthcare disparities among orthopedic trauma patients in the USA: socio-demographic factors influence the management of calcaneus fractures. J Orthop Surg Res 2019;14(1):359.
38. Schairer WW, Nwachukwu BU, Warren RF, et al. Operative Fixation for Clavicle Fractures-Socioeconomic Differences Persist Despite Overall Population Increases in Utilization. J Orthop Trauma 2017;31(6):e167–72.
39. Collins JE, Katz JN, Donnell-Fink LA, et al. Cumulative incidence of ACL reconstruction after ACL injury in adults. AJSM 2013;41:544–9.
40. Bram JT, Talathi NS, Patel NM, et al. How Do Race and Insurance Status Affect the Care of Pediatric Anterior Cruciate Ligament Injuries? Clin J Sport Med 2020;30(6):e201-e206.
41. Hwang A, Zhang L, Ramirez G, et al. Black Race, Hispanic Ethnicity, and Medicaid Insurance Are Associated With Lower Rates of Rotator Cuff Repair in New York State. Arthroscopy 2022;38(11):3001–10.e2.
42. Farley KX, Dawes AM, Wilson JM, et al. Racial Disparities in the Utilization of Shoulder Arthroplasty in the United States: Trends from 2011 to 2017. JB JS Open Access 2022;7(2):e21.00144.
43. Wallace J, Covassin T, Moran R. Racial Disparities in Concussion Knowledge and Symptom Recognition in American Adolescent Athletes. J Racial Ethn Health Disparities 2018;5(1):221–8.
44. McCrory P, Meeuwisse WH, Aubry M, et al. Consensus statement on concussion in sport: the 4th International Conference on Concussion in Sport, Zurich, November 2012. J Athl Train 2013;48(4):554–75.
45. McLendon LA, Kralik SF, Grayson PA, et al. The controversial second impact syndrome: A review of the literature. Pediatr Neurol 2016;62:9–17.
46. Lyons TW, Miller KA, Miller AF, Mannix R. Racial and Ethnic Differences in Emergency Department Utilization and Diagnosis for Sports-Related Head Injuries. Front Neurol 2019;10:690.

47. Kontos AP, Elbin RJ 3rd, Covassin T, Larson E. Exploring differences in computerized neurocognitive concussion testing between African American and White athletes. Arch Clin Neuropsychol 2010;25(8):734–44.
48. Eagle SR, Brent D, Covassin T, et al. Exploration of Race and Ethnicity, Sex, Sport-Related Concussion, Depression History, and Suicide Attempts in US Youth. JAMA Netw Open 2022;5(7):e2219934.
49. The Associated Press. The NFL wills top assuming racial differences when assessing brain injuries. NPR. Published June 2, 2021 Available at: https://www.npr.org/2021/06/02/1002627309/nfl-says-it-will-halt-race-norming-and-review-brain-injury-claims. Accessed August 1, 2022.
50. The Associated Press. Judge approves fix to stem race bias in NFL concussion deal. Published March 4, 2022 Available at: https://www.nfl.com/news/judge-approves-fix-to-stem-race-bias-in-nfl-concussion-deal. Accessed May 27, 2023.
51. The Associated Press. Judge approves fix to stem race bias in NFL concussion deal. Published March 4, 2022 Available at: https://www.nfl.com/news/judge-approves-fix-to-stem-race-bias-in-nfl-concussion-deal. Accessed May 27, 2023.
52. Dickason RM, Chauhan V, Mor A, et al. Racial differences in opiate administration for pain relief at an academic emergency department. West J Emerg Med 2015;16(3):372–80.
53. Goyal MK, Kuppermann N, Cleary SD, et al. Racial disparities in pain management of children with appendicitis in emergency departments. JAMA Pediatr 2015;169:996–1002.
54. Hollingshead NA, Meints SM, Miller MM, et al. A comparison of race-related pain stereotypes held by White and Black individuals. J Appl Soc Psychol 2016;46(12):718–23.
55. Dore RA, Hoffman KM, Lillard AS, Trawalter S. Children's racial bias in perceptions of others' pain. Br J Dev Psychol 2014;32(2):218–31.
56. Trawalter S, Hoffman KM, Waytz A. Racial bias in perceptions of other's pain. PLoS One 2012;7(11):e48546 1–8.
57. Druckman JN, Trawalter S, Montes I, et al. Racial bias in sport medical staff's perceptions of other's pain. J Soc Psychol 2018;158(6):721–9.
58. Butts HF. Economic Stress and Mental Health. J Natl Med Assoc 1979;71(4):375–9.
59. Black A, Woods-Giscombe C. Applying the stress and "strength" hypothesis to Black women's breast cancer screening delays. Stress Health 2012;28(5):389–96.
60. Barnnes DM, Bates LM. Do racial patterns in psychological distress shed light on the Black-White depression paradox? A systematic review. Soc Psychiatry Psychiatr Epidemil 2017;52(8):913–28.
61. Williams DR. Stress and the mental health of populations of color: advancing our understanding of race-related stressors. J Health Soc Behav 2018;59(4):466–85.
62. McClendon J, Chang K, Boudreaux MJ, et al. Black-White racial health disparities in inflammation and physical health: Cumulative stress, social isolation, and health behaviors. Psychoneuroendocrinology 2021;131:105251.
63. Adelani MA, O'Connor MI. Perspectives of orthopaedic surgeons on racial/ethnic disparities in care. J Racial and Ethninc Disparities 2017;4(4):758–62.
64. Tajfel H, Turner JC. An integrative theory of inter-group conflict. In: Austin WG, Worchel S, editors. The social psychology of Inter-group Relations. Monterey, CA: Brooks/Cole; 1979. p. 33–47.
65. Stephan WS, Stephan CW. An integrated threat theory of prejudice. Reducing prejudice and discrimination. New York: Psychology Press; 2013. p. 33–56.

66. Byrne D. Interpersonal attraction and attitude similarity. J Abnorm Soc Psychol 1961;62:713–5.
67. Byrne D, Wong TJ. Racial prejudice, interpersonal attraction, and assumed dissimilarity of attitudes. J of Abnormal and Social Psychology 1962;65(4): 246–53.
68. Chornokur G, Dalton K, Borysova ME, et al. Disparities at presentation, diagnosis, treatment, and survival in African American men, affected by prostate cancer. Prostate 2011;71(9):985–97.
69. Cooper LA, Roter DL, Johnson RL, et al. Patient-centered communication, ratings of care, and concordance of patient and physician race. Ann Intern Med 2003; 139:907–15.
70. Cooper-Patrick L, Gallo JJ, Gonzales JJ, et al. Race, gender, and partnership in the patient-physician relationship. JAMA 1999;282(6):583–9.
71. Saha S, Beach MC. Impact of physician race on patient decision making and ratings of physicians: a randomized experiment using video vignettes. J Gen Intern Med 2020;35(4):1084–91.
72. Shen MJ, Peterson EB, Costas-Muñiz R, et al. The Effects of Race and Racial Concordance on Patient-Physician Communication: A Systematic Review of the Literature. J Racial Ethn Health Disparities 2018;5(1):117–40.
73. Tobin MJ. Fiftieth anniversary of uncovering the Tuskegee Syphilis Study: The story and timeless lessons. Am J Respir Crit Care Med 2022;205(10):1145–58.
74. Wall LL. The medical ethics of Dr. J Marion Sims: a fresh look at the historical record. J Med Ethics 2006;32(6):346–50.
75. Baptiste DL, Caviness-Ashe N, Josiah N, et al. Henrietta Lacks and America's dark history of research involving African Americans. Nurs Open 2022;9(5): 2236–8.
76. Ku L, Vichare A. The association of racial and ethnic concordance in primary care with patient satisfaction and experience of care. J Gen Intern Med 2023;38(3): 272–332.
77. Bai X, Ramos MR, Fiske ST. As diversity increases, people paradoxically perceive social groups as more similar. Proc Natl Acad Sci USA 2020;117(23):12741–9.
78. Crisp RJ, Turner RN. Cognitive adaptation to the experience of social and cultural diversity. Psychol Bull 2011;137:242–66.
79. Schmid K, Hewstone M, Ramiah AA. Neighborhood diversity and social identity complexity: implications for intergroup relations. Soc Psychol Personal Sci 2013;4:135–42.

Section II: What can we do

Diversity in Orthopaedic Surgery: What Is Next? What is Needed Collectively? How Do You Go About Effecting Positive Change?

Jason L. Koh, MD, MBA[a,b,*]

KEYWORDS

• Diversity • Orthopedic surgery • Pipeline • Gender • Ethnicity • Inclusion

KEY POINTS

- Orthopedic surgery as a field is the least diverse medical specialty.
- Multiple factors contribute to the lack of diversity, including lack of diversity in medical school, lack of role models and mentors, and discrimination and bias.
- Addressing the lack of diversity includes use of data, implementation of targeted pipeline programs, individual physician advocacy, institutional recruitment and DEI initiatives, and leadership from professional organizations.
- Targeted pipeline programs and role models and mentors are very effective in increasing diversity.

WHAT IS NEXT

The United States is a diverse country and becoming more so with time. In addition, more dimensions of diversity are increasingly recognized. Census data show that racial and ethnic diversity will continue to increase, and the Census Bureau has predicted by 2045 that the United States will have no single race or ethnicity as the majority.[1] In addition, the number of women in medicine continues to increase to the point where they compromise the majority of students entering medical school classes as of 2019.[2]

Conversely, orthopedic surgery remains one of the least diverse medical specialties in terms of race, ethnicity, and gender diversity. According to the 2022 Association of

---

No relevant financial disclosures.

[a] Orthopaedic & Spine Institute; [b] NorthShore University HealthSystem, Illinois, University of Chicago Pritzker School of Medicine
* 9669 North Kenton Avenue, Suite 406, Skokie, IL 60076.
E-mail address: drjasonkoh@gmail.com

Clin Sports Med 43 (2024) 245–251
https://doi.org/10.1016/j.csm.2023.06.021

American Medical Colleges (AAMC) Physician Specialty Data Report orthopedic surgery has the fewest representation of active Hispanic identifying physicians (3.3%) and one of the lowest percentage of Black identifying physicians (3.2%). Overall, orthopedic surgery has the highest of white identifying physicians of any specialty (83.6%). The percentage of women orthopedic surgeons is 5.9%, which is the lowest percentage of any specialty.[3] The percentage of women is somewhat higher in orthopedic sports medicine, with the gender distribution of sports fellows averaging 11.4% women during 2016 to 2021.[4] Nevertheless, these numbers are striking because other surgical fields have been significantly more successful in addressing issues of diversity. For example, the 2022 general surgery applicant pool was 50.7% women, as opposed to orthopedic surgery, which was 23.7%.[5] Change can clearly occur, but it has been much slower in orthopedic surgery.

This lack of diversity has implications for patient care, as research has identified that diversity in health care teams leads to better patient outcomes, including increased patient satisfaction and improved quality of care.[6–8] Patients from underrepresented minority groups may feel more comfortable obtaining care from physicians with similar backgrounds.[9] A diverse workforce has been demonstrated to have improved performance, and different perspectives can lead to more creative and effective solutions for complex problems.[10] Minority researchers may promote additional research into health care disparities.[11] In addition, minority physicians are more likely to work in underserved areas.[12–14]

What Is Needed Collectively?

There are many factors that result in the lack of diversity in orthopedic surgery and sports medicine. The pathway to orthopedic surgery has multiple barriers, starting with college and medical school admissions and extending to orthopedic residency and fellowship programs.[15] For example, there remains a lack of racial diversity in medical school students.[5] A lack of role models and mentors plays an important role in choice of career. Students from underrepresented groups often face financial and social barriers to entry, such as higher student loan debt and lack of access to professional networks. Discrimination and bias (both conscious and unconscious) discourage students from applying to orthopedic residency programs. Even after acceptance into programs, discrimination can continue, along with microaggressions and harassment that can result in departure from residency.[16] Finally, orthopedic leadership remains essentially Caucasian and male, with few exceptions at the faculty and organizational level.[17,18]

In order to address the lack of diversity, equity, and inclusion in orthopedic surgery and sports medicine, there are several key steps that can be taken. In general, these steps include increasing recognition of the scope and importance of the issue; building supportive environments that are free from discrimination and bias, and outreach and recruitment. Specific measures include increasing representation of underrepresented groups at every stage of the pipeline, from medical school admissions to residency and fellowship positions, and into faculty and leadership positions, creating a culture of inclusion through support and training, and offering mentorship and sponsorship opportunities for underrepresented groups.

How Do You Go About Effecting Positive Change?

There are multiple strategies that can be used to create positive change. One key aspect is to create awareness of the problem by identifying and publicizing data around the lack of diversity in orthopedic surgery. By tracking diversity metrics and analyzing the data, orthopedic surgery groups can identify areas of improvement and implement targeted interventions to address disparities. Consciously bringing attention to these metrics stimulates problem solving and action to address these issues. These metrics can also be used to highlight programs that have been successful in actively improving diversity, which provide examples to the larger orthopedic community. In addition, cross-specialty comparison can heighten the recognition that orthopedics in this area significantly trails other specialties. For example, even specialties that have traditionally been male-dominated such as general surgery now have majority female applicants to residency. The data-demonstrated success of different groups is a powerful message that positive change can be achieved despite obstacles.

Another technique is the implementation of targeted pipeline programs that specifically address the needs of underrepresented groups. The pathway to orthopedic surgery is long and challenging, and orthopedic surgery is one of the most competitive medical specialties to match for residency. Most successful applicants, in addition to having excellent academic records, have strong sponsorship and support as well as often having participated in additional research. Students from underrepresented groups may be as familiar with the common preparation involved in applying to competitive residencies, such as participating in research, or may not have access or financial resources to take advantage of these types of opportunities. Without mentors, they may not have guidance in navigating this pathway.

One example of a pipeline program is the Perry Initiative, which aims to increase female representation in orthopedic surgery by targeting women in high school and in medical school and has been successful in reaching more than 13,000 students since 2009.[19] This group has several programs that introduce women to role models, mentors, and surgical procedures in the area of orthopedics.

Another example is Nth Dimensions, which is one of the most successful pipeline programs in the United States for women and minorities seeking competitive specialties.[20,21] Founded in 2004 by Dr Bonnie Simpson-Mason, an African-American woman orthopedic surgeon, the mission is to “eliminate health care disparities in all communities by diversifying the physician workforce.” This organization sponsors bioskills workshops, summer internship programs, and medical student symposiums aimed at undergraduate and medical school students, as well as continuing mentorship, coaching, and advice. The results are phenomenal, with female Nth Dimensions Scholars 45x more likely to apply to orthopedic residency[21,22] and an average 92% match rate for the past 5 years. This program has clearly shown the benefit of a focused pipeline program.

Individual Strategies

Individual physicians and surgeons can play a crucial role in effecting positive change by committing to diversity and being allied to underrepresented groups; this begins by education and recognition of the impact of racism and sexism on the field. Self-examination and reflection about conscious and unconscious bias and the relative advantages and disadvantages of different groups helps build awareness and provides an opportunity to change thought and behavior. Physicians can create a more inclusive and welcoming culture in orthopedic surgery and sports medicine through many ways, including speaking up when discriminatory statements or action occurs. They can actively seek out opportunities to learn from and collaborate with individuals from diverse backgrounds, including serving as formal or informal mentors.

In addition, individuals can advocate for DEI initiatives within their own practices, groups, and medical facilities. These initiatives include working to recruit diverse candidates, providing mentorship and development opportunities to underrepresented minority groups, implementing training programs, and promoting diversity in leadership positions. They can also serve as important allies within their organizations as well as support professional organizations such as the Ruth Jackson Orthopaedic Society or the J. Robert Gladden Orthopaedic Society that promote increasing the diversity within orthopedic surgery.

Institutional Strategies

Institutions such as medical schools, residency and fellowship programs, and hospitals and health care systems play an important role in effecting positive change. Medical schools play a critical early role in the preparation and training of the next generation of orthopedic surgeons. To address the lack of diversity, medical schools need to actively recruit and support students from underrepresented groups by providing mentorship, financial and academic support, and other resources to ensure that students can be successful in their training. DEI training can help create a more inclusive culture.

In addition, medical schools and training programs need to specifically recruit and retain diverse faculty and promote an inclusive culture. Specific recruiting strategies can deliberately seek out diverse individuals and expand the pool of candidates for positions, similar to the "Rooney Rule" in the NFL. Highlighting role models and the importance of DEI initiatives within an organization can also help with recruiting and retaining diverse individuals. The impact of role models and URM representation on developing the pipeline is well established. Higher URM representation among orthopedic faculty increases orthopedic residency application among medical students (odds ratio 1.27). Even more striking is the effect of high URM representation in residency programs, where URM student residency application rates were 45% higher than in other programs.[23] Similar effects have been seen with increased female medical students applying for orthopedic surgery who attend school at institutions with higher resident and faculty gender diversity.[24] Women are more likely than men to state that same-sex role models positively influenced their choice to pursue orthopedics,[25] and so female faculty participation is very important.

Within an institution, a supportive structure is critical for the retention of diverse individuals. Efforts should be made to address implicit bias and microaggressions. A strategy that is supportive of appropriate work-life balance including accommodations for pregnancy, childbirth, nursing, and childcare is very helpful to attract faculty. Mentorship and promotion to leadership positions for diverse individuals are also important.

Hospitals and health care systems also have an important role in addressing the lack of diversity in orthopedic surgery. These organizations can actively recruit and retain staff and physicians of diverse backgrounds. They can support DEI initiatives, including training in cultural competency, implicit bias, and effective communication with patients from diverse backgrounds. In addition, just as in academic centers, mentorship and promotion to leadership of diverse individuals plays an important role.

Professional Organizations

Professional organizations play a vital role in shaping the direction of the field. Smaller groups focused on diversity issues such as the Ruth Jackson Orthopaedic Society (women) and the J. Robert Gladden Orthopaedic Society (URM) play important roles in providing mentors and role models to diverse students, residents, fellows, and practitioners. Specific programs, such as the scholarships provided to medical students to attend the Ruth Jackson meeting, can have a powerful impact. For example, 80% of the women who were scholarship recipients became active in orthopedics as opposed to the 45% who did not.[26] Larger organizations that represent more general groups of orthopedic surgeons such as the American Academy of Orthopaedic Surgeons (AAOS), the American Orthopaedic Society for Sports Medicine (AOSSM), and the International Society of Arthroscopy, Knee Surgery and Orthopaedic Sports Medicine (ISAKOS) also can have a leadership role in promoting DEI. These organizations can work to provide training, mentorship, and outreach to underrepresented groups. The AAOS has had a strong commitment to diversity, with the Diversity Advisory Board (DAB) playing a role in overseeing all activities of the AAOS. It produces an annual scorecard and actively seeks to promote diversity in its committee and leadership structure. AAOS leadership actively supports diversity and speaks frequently to educate and advocate for increased diversity. This message is further carried forward by symposia, research articles and publications, and through the AAOS Now newsletter and other media outlets. The AAOS Diversity Award is one of the most prominent recognitions of the importance of DEI. AOSSM initiated a DEI Task Force in 2021 to explore issues related to diversity and develop strategies to address them. Recently (2023) the AOSSM Board approved the creation of a DEI Committee, with ex officio representation on the board of the organization and involvement with various committees. Similarly, in 2021 ISAKOS launched a Gender Diversity Task Force, which has successfully had several webinars, recruited additional female members (nearly doubling the number), and helped place women in the committee structure and promoted significantly more participation in podium talks, panels, and symposia.

Orthopedic Community

Finally, the orthopedic community at large has a critical role in addressing the lack of DEI in the field, which includes working to actively promote and support DEI initiatives, such as mentorship programs, diversity and inclusion training, and outreach to underrepresented minority groups.

In addition, the orthopedic community can work to create a more welcoming and inclusive culture; this includes actively promoting and supporting staff and physicians from diverse backgrounds, creating safe spaces for patients and staff from underrepresented minority groups, and actively working to address implicit biases that may exist within the field. We all have a role in shaping the culture of orthopedic surgery.

SUMMARY

As the United States becomes a more diverse country, it is even more important that the orthopedic community evolves to reflect this diversity and provide the highest quality of care. Unfortunately, orthopedic surgery remains the least diverse of all of the medical specialties. We need to increase recognition of the scope and importance of the issue, build supportive environments that are free from discrimination and bias, and promote outreach and recruitment at all levels from middle and high school students to the highest levels of leadership. Fortunately, individuals and groups can make a substantive difference through multiple ways including changing the culture, creating pipeline programs, and promoting diverse individuals. We are consciously addressing these issues, and already there is clear evidence that the future orthopedic workforce will be more diverse. Change can and will occur.

CLINICS CARE POINTS

- Diversity in health care teams leads to better outcomes.

- Multiple factors for the lack of diversity in orthopaedics include lack of racial diversity in medical students, lack of role models, and bias (including unconscious) that discourages students.
- Pipeline programs and role models are effective in increasing diveristy in orthopaedic surgery.

REFERENCES

1. Frey W. The nation is diversifying even faster than predicted, according to new census data. Washington DC: Brookings; 2020. p. 2020.
2. Association of American Medical Colleges. 2019 Fall applicant, matriculant, and enrollment data tables. Washington, DC: Association of American Medical Colleges; 2019.
3. 2022 Physician specialty data report. Association of American Medical Colleges; 2022.
4. Kamalapathy P, Moore A, Brockmeier S, et al. Status quo: trends in diversity and unique traits among orthopaedic sports medicine fellowship directors. J Am Acad Orthop Surg 2022;30(1):36–43.
5. Curtin L.S.G.R., Lamb D.L., Applicant Demographics and the Transition to Residency: It's Time to Leverage Data on Preferred Specialty and Match Outcomes to Inform the National Conversation about Diversity and Equity in Medical Education. Available at: https://www.nrmp.org/wp-content/uploads/2023/02/Demographic-data-perspectives-paper_FINAL.pdf. Accessed April 26, 2023.
6. Alsan MGO, Graziani G. Does diversity matter for health? Experimental evidence from Oakland. Am Econ Rev 2019;109(12):4071–111.
7. Arvizo C, Garrison E. Diversity and inclusion: the role of unconscious bias on patient care, health outcomes and the workforce in obstetrics and gynaecology. Curr Opin Obstet Gynecol 2019;31(5):356–62.
8. Logghe H, Jones C, McCoubrey A, et al. #ILookLikeASurgeon: embracing diversity to improve patient outcomes. BMJ 2017;359:j4653.
9. Wright MA, Murthi AM, Aleem A, et al. Patient disparities and provider diversity in orthopaedic surgery: a complex relationship. J Am Acad Orthop Surg 2023; 31(3):132–9.
10. Gomez LE, Bernet P. Diversity improves performance and outcomes. J Natl Med Assoc 2019;111(4):383–92.
11. Wallington SF, Dash C, Sheppard VB, et al. Enrolling minority and underserved populations in cancer clinical research. Am J Prev Med 2016;50(1):111–7.
12. Phelan SM, Burke SE, Cunningham BA, et al. The effects of racism in medical education on students' decisions to practice in underserved or minority communities. Acad Med 2019;94(8):1178–89.
13. Marrast LM, Zallman L, Woolhandler S, et al. Minority physicians' role in the care of underserved patients: diversifying the physician workforce may be key in addressing health disparities. JAMA Intern Med 2014;174(2):289–91.
14. Cerasani M, Omoruan M, Rieber C, et al. Demographic factors and medical school experiences associated with students' intention to pursue orthopaedic surgery and practice in underserved areas, *JB JS Open Access*, 8 (1):e22.00016, 2023, 1-8.
15. Lamanna DL, Chen AF, Dyer GSM, et al. Diversity and inclusion in orthopaedic surgery from medical school to practice: AOA critical issues. J Bone Joint Surg Am 2022;104(18):e80.

16. Brooks JT, Porter SE, Middleton KK, et al. The majority of black orthopaedic surgeons report experiencing racial microaggressions during their residency training. Clin Orthop Relat Res 2023;481(4):675–86.
17. Julian KR, Anand M, Sobel AD, et al. A 5-year update and comparison of factors related to the sex diversity of orthopaedic residency programs in the United States, *JB JS Open Access*, 8 (1):e22.00116, 2023, 1-5.
18. Shah KN, Ruddell JH, Scott B, et al. Orthopaedic Surgery Faculty: An Evaluation of Gender and Racial Diversity Compared with Other Specialties. JB JS. Open Access 2022;5(3):e20.00009.
19. The Perry Initiative: Building the Pipeline for Women in Engineering and Medicine 2023. Available at: https://perryinitiative.org/. Accessed April 26, 2023.
20. Nth Dimensions 2023. Updated 2023. Available at: https://www.nthdimensions.org/. Accessed April 26, 2023.
21. Mason BS, Ross W, Ortega G, et al. Can a strategic pipeline initiative increase the number of women and underrepresented minorities in orthopaedic surgery? Clin Orthop Relat Res 2016;474(9):1979–85.
22. Mason B, Ross WAJ Jr, Bradford L. Nth dimensions evolution, impact, and recommendations for equity practices in orthopaedics. J Am Acad Orthop Surg 2022; 30(8):350–7.
23. Okike K, Phillips DP, Johnson WA, et al. Orthopaedic faculty and resident racial/ethnic diversity is associated with the orthopaedic application rate among underrepresented minority medical students. J Am Acad Orthop Surg 2020;28(6): 241–7.
24. Okike K, Phillips DP, Swart E, et al. Orthopaedic faculty and resident sex diversity are associated with the orthopaedic residency application rate of female medical students. J Bone Joint Surg Am 2019;101(12):e56.
25. Hill JF, Yule A, Zurakowski D, et al, Day CS. Residents' perceptions of sex diversity in orthopaedic surgery. J Bone Joint Surg Am 2013;95(19):e1441–6.
26. Vajapey S, Cannada LK, Samora JB. What proportion of women who received funding to attend a ruth jackson orthopaedic society meeting pursued a career in orthopaedics? Clin Orthop Relat Res 2019;477(7):1722–6.

Strengthening the Pipeline

Promoting Diversity into Orthopedic Surgery

Maike van Niekerk, PhD, Alana O'Mara, BS, Stephanie Kha, MD, Joanne Zhou, MD, Timothy A. McAdams, MD, Amy Ladd, MD, Kevin Shea, MD, Steven Frick, MD, William J. Maloney, MD, Constance R. Chu, MD*

KEYWORDS

• Diversity • Equity • Orthopedic surgery • Mentorship • Team physician

KEY POINTS

- Orthopedic surgery shows severe underrepresentation of women and minority populations at the resident, fellow, attending, and team physician levels.
- Underrepresentation in orthopedic surgery is a multifactorial problem perpetuated throughout the pipeline, with common barriers including deep-rooted stereotypes, limited clinical exposure and mentorship, and exclusive work environments.
- Several organizations have been established around the world in order to promote diversity in orthopedic surgery, offering mentorship, educational initiatives, and career advancement opportunities for a variety of groups, including women, racial and ethnic minorities, and people in the lesbian, gay, bisexual, transgender, and queer + community.
- Stanford University and orthopedic faculty have developed and implemented pipeline approaches, which include early musculoskeletal didactic and clinical experiences, mentorship and research programs, and a demonstrated commitment to recruiting and retaining individuals from diverse backgrounds.
- Broader implementation of pipeline programs to improve diversity at every stage of professional development from high school to leadership positions is needed to improve diversity in orthopedic surgery and among orthopedic team physicians.

INTRODUCTION

When Pittsburgh Steeler's head team physician James Bradley was asked by management why he wanted Craig Bennett to be his assistant team physician, he replied, "because he is the best person for the job." When asked the same question a few years later when he nominated Robin West for the same position, he replied, "because she is the best person for the job" (James Bradley, M.D. and Constance Chu, MD, e-mail, July 22, 2022). Both historic choices were approved with Drs Bennett and

Department of Orthopedic Surgery, Stanford University, Stanford, CA, USA
* Corresponding author.
E-mail address: chucr@stanford.edu

Clin Sports Med 43 (2024) 253–270
https://doi.org/10.1016/j.csm.2023.07.007
sportsmed.theclinics.com

West becoming, respectively, the first African American and the first female assistant team physicians for the franchise. Twenty-five years later, Dr. Bennett remains 1 of just 2 African Americans and Dr. West 1 of just 2 women orthopedic surgeons to have served the *National Football League* (*NFL*) as team physicians. Becoming a team physician for a professional sports organization is a highly competitive multi-tier process requiring mentorship and sponsorship by established team physicians. Prerequisites include matriculation and graduation from medical school, distinguishing oneself to secure a highly competitive orthopedic surgery residency and an orthopedic sports medicine fellowship, and succeeding at mentored experience caring for professional teams and athletes. Board certification requires an additional 2 years of operative patient care passing rigorous written and oral examinations. This is an arduous climb occupying at least 12 years after graduation from college.

Athletes represent the full spectrum of the nation's population. In several popular sports, minority populations predominate at the elite and professional levels. All genders participate in sports whether actively or as fans and supporters. However, the orthopedic surgeons who serve as team physicians are Caucasian and male with staggeringly few exceptions.

Improving diversity among qualified orthopedic team physicians is a long and overdue process that starts with enhancing diversity within orthopedic surgery. In 2018, more than 90% of practicing orthopedic surgeons reported themselves to be male and Caucasian.[1] Despite improvements in representation, the pace of progress has been noticeably slower than in other medical and surgical specialties.[1] In the United States, 18% of the active orthopedic surgery residents identify as female, 5% as Black or African American, and 7% as Hispanic, Latino, or Spanish origin, with the proportions being even lower among attendings.[1,2] Compared with each group's prevalence in the United States, such statistics demonstrate a mismatch.[1,3] This article highlights ongoing and emerging strategies to engage, mentor, and sponsor members of underrepresented groups to successfully become the best person for the job of an orthopedic team physician.

Disparities in orthopedic patient care among women and racial and ethnic minorities may be linked, at least in part, to limited diversity in their providers. Patients who identify with their physicians have better outcomes, including improved physician-patient interactions, greater adherence to treatments, and faster recovery.[4] Previous studies have found that sex-discordance between surgeons and patients may be associated with greater adverse postoperative outcomes.[5] Additionally, physicians from minority backgrounds are more likely to practice in underserved areas, thereby providing much-needed access to care to overlooked patient populations.[1]

In response to the importance of improving diversity in orthopedic surgery, a number of non-profit organizations, academic institutions, and orthopedic societies have developed initiatives aimed at addressing equity and inclusion in the field.[1,6] Many of these initiatives offer students, residents, fellows, and attendings with mentorship opportunities, educational seminars, research grants, academic scholarships, and events showcasing orthopedic surgeons from diverse backgrounds. This manuscript provides an overview of the current landscape of diversity in orthopedic surgery, discusses barriers, and summarizes pipeline initiatives at one academic institution that can be further developed by other institutions to enhance diversity in orthopedic surgery.

CURRENT LANDSCAPE

Currently, orthopedics has the lowest percentage of female physicians of all specialties (**Fig. 1**).[2,7–12] In the National Graduate Medical Education (GME) Census report

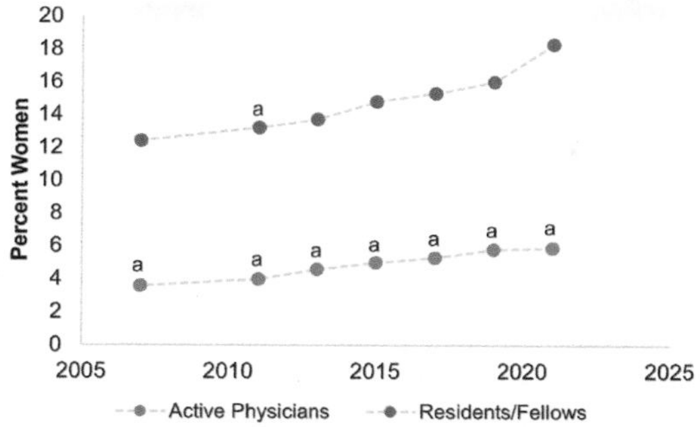

Fig. 1. National GME Census GME track reports on percentage of female practicing orthopedic surgeons.[2,7–12]Acronym: GME, Graduate Medical Education.[a] Represents the lowest percentage of 48 medical and surgical specialties.

from 2021, only 5.9% of the orthopedic surgeons and 18.3% of the trainees were women.[12] Despite the limited diversity, orthopedic surgery has been slow to change. From 2012 to 2020, women's representation went up by a mere 3.3%; this is in comparison to other surgical specialties, such as plastic surgery, which showed an increase in women by 12%.[13] Similarly, the representation of minorities lags in orthopedics (**Fig. 2**).[14–16] This pattern extends to leadership positions within academic settings, national organizations, and editorial positions in top orthopedic journals.[17] Only 9 women have been orthopedic department chairs in the United States,[17] and African American and Hispanic orthopedic surgeons of both sexes are underrepresented at all levels of clinical and academic orthopedics.[3] Additionally, women make up less than 10% of the editorial boards in the top orthopedic journals, compared with 21% in general surgery journals and 35% in internal medicine journals.[18]

BARRIERS TO DIVERSITY

Improving diversity in orthopedic surgery is a multifactorial, complex issue. Underrepresentation is perpetuated throughout the pipeline of training and professional development in orthopedic surgery.[3] Previous literature has proposed that the "bottleneck" for improving orthopedic surgery diversity appears to reside at the medical school level.[19] Deep-rooted stereotypes, limited early exposure, limited access to mentors, and exclusive work environments are commonly cited barriers to improving representation in this field.[20–23]

Deep-Rooted Stereotypes

Deep-rooted stereotypes about orthopedic surgery are a significant barrier to improving diversification in orthopedic surgery. It is perceived by many that Caucasian males are overwhelmingly dominant, thereby discouraging those who do not fit into this stereotype.[6] Such stereotypes are reinforced by statistics regarding the limited diversity among orthopedic surgery residents and attendings.[17] In the absence of adequate exposure, students may struggle to form their own independent views of the field. Previous literature has found that before orthopedic clinical rotations, women are less likely than men to agree that diversity and inclusion are an integral part of the orthopedic culture.[20] However, clinical rotations often change students' perceptions. After clinical rotations, women were significantly more likely to believe that diversity and inclusion are a part of the orthopedic surgery culture, and that orthopedic surgery is friendlier, more diverse, and more inclusive.[20]

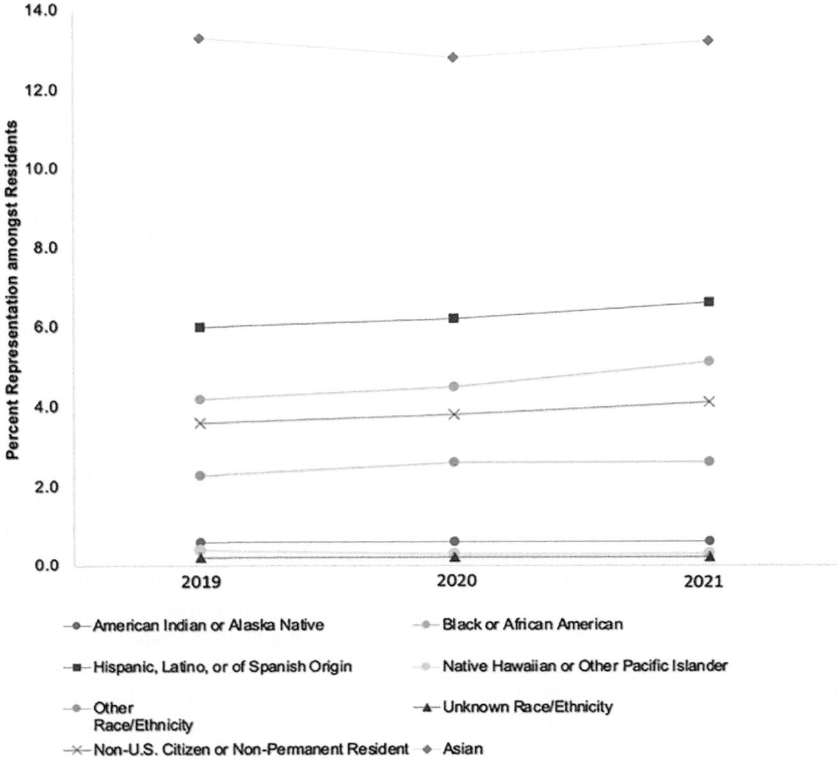

Fig. 2. Percentage of minorities among resident physicians in orthopedics, divided by entering year[14–16].

Limited Early Exposure

In light of the findings outlined previously, it is imperative that medical students gain early exposure to orthopedic surgery.[24] Yet, nearly half of medical schools in the United States do not offer a musculoskeletal (MSK) curriculum and only 15% require an MSK rotation, with some institutions having no orthopedic programs at all, leaving many medical students with limited exposure to orthopedic surgery at an early stage.[3] Diverse applicants are disproportionately affected by this limited exposure. Unlike male students who have been found to be significantly more likely to choose orthopedic surgery before entering clinical rotations (with twice the rate of wishing to enter the field *prior* to medical school compared with female students), women are more likely to choose it as a career after clinical exposures and elective experiences.[25] Perhaps unsurprisingly, women who attend medical schools with mandatory MSK curricula were found to be 75% more likely to apply to orthopedic surgery residency programs than those who did not,[6] and implementation of orthopedic surgery rotations has been associated with an 81% increase in female applicants and 101% increase in minorities.[26]

Despite the potential that clinical rotations hold in improving representation in the field, it is important to acknowledge that students who develop an interest in orthopedic surgery after clinical rotations have less time to strengthen their application to become competitive applicants, creating another barrier to entry in the absence of additional earlier mechanisms of exposure. It is therefore important to consider exposure at earlier stages, such as at the level of high school or college.

Sports participation, spectatorship, and cultivation of team spirit are integral to high school and college experiences for many students. This provides potential opportunities to develop programs to expose women and minority students to sports medicine. For example, institutions can pair students from minority backgrounds with team physicians, athletic trainers, and physical therapists in their freshman year to provide them with exposure, knowledge, and experience in sports medicine.

Limited Access to Mentors and Role Models

Along with early exposure to orthopedic surgery and sports medicine, mentorship is also critical to success. A lack of reliable mentorship or representation of faculty from minority backgrounds is cited as a common barrier to increasing diversity in orthopedics.[24,27] The importance of mentorship is particularly evident for underrepresented groups, where a greater proportion of women (59%) than men (25%) have stated that having a role model of a similar ethnicity or gender is a positive factor in their decision to enter orthopedic surgery.[28] A study of recently-matched underrepresented minority students similarly found that the vast majority of students (89%) indicated that the presence or absence of underrepresented minority faculty influenced their rank list.[29] Further, women who attend medical schools with higher sex diversity among orthopedic faculty and residents have been found to be significantly more likely to apply to orthopedic surgery residency programs (Odds Ratio [OR] = 1.30, $P < .05$).[23] Given the aforementioned effects of mentorships, longitudinal mentoring programs can be implemented at all career stages of orthopedic surgery to promote a pipeline of inclusivity.

Exclusive Work Environments

Exclusive work environments documented in orthopedic surgery and sports medicine can act as deterrents for medical students considering a career in the field and can lead to attrition of residents, fellows, and attendings. Microaggressions are unfortunately pervasive in orthopedic surgery, with 3 in 4 female orthopedic surgeons experiencing them during their training.[30] Such experiences, while seemingly trivial, can undermine relationships, compromise quality of care, lower self-esteem, and cause psychological distress, potentially dissuade women from pursuing this career, and prevent women from achieving their potential in orthopedic surgery.[31] Additionally, women are more likely to experience bullying, harassment, and sexual abuse.[22,31] A recent survey of *Ruth Jackson Orthopedic Society* members demonstrated that over two-thirds of the respondents had experienced sexual harassment during their orthopedic residency training, with no improvements found between current and past trainees.[21] Prior studies have reported similar estimates that half of women experience sexual harassment during their careers, compared with 10% of men.[22]

Orthopedic surgery residency applicants from underrepresented backgrounds are also subjected to bias and discrimination, including inappropriate, gender-biased questions during residency interviews. There are reports that 3 in 5 female orthopedic surgery applicants are asked such questions, with no improvement found over 5 decades.[32] These questions often focus on marital status (24% females vs 7% males queried), family planning (61% females vs 8% males queried), and children (33% females vs 4% males queried).[33] Women have been found to be less likely to rank programs that ask these questions,[33] likely leading to reductions in the diversity of the cohorts of incoming orthopedic residents. These biased and discriminatory behaviors, despite being illegal, often go unreported out of fear of negative consequences and are therefore perpetuated.[32] In addition, outside of departmental bias, oftentimes bias from other services or ancillary staff can be a source of moral injury.[34]

Discrimination against racial and ethnic minorities also exists in this field. Approximately 97% of respondents in a recent survey of Black orthopedic surgeons in the United States believed that Black orthopedic surgeons face workplace discrimination, with Black female surgeons reporting higher levels of discrimination and lower occupational opportunities than Black male surgeons.[35] These findings come in conjunction with recent literature suggesting that unrepresented minority residents represent 17.5% of all residents who resigned or were dismissed, while representing only 6% of all residents during that same period.[27]

DIVERSITY, EQUITY, AND INCLUSION (DEI) INITIATIVES

DEI Organizations

Several organizations have been established in the United States and worldwide to promote the diversification of orthopedic surgery, some of which are summarized in **Table 1**. Diverse groups are targeted by these organizations, including women,[36–39,44] racial and ethnic minorities,[38,40,41,44] and members of the lesbian, gay, bisexual, transgender, and queer (LGBTQ+)community.[43] Despite the fact that each organization has its own unique focus, many offer mentorship programs,[36–38,40,41,43,44] facilitate educational initiatives,[31,36-41,43-45] and provide research awards and travel grants to help individuals navigate orthopedic surgery and advance their careers.[36,37,40,41,43,44]

The Ruth Jackson Orthopedic Society, established in 1983, is perhaps the earliest organization dedicated to improving diversity in the field.[36] With over 1400 members of female orthopedic surgeons, residents, fellows, medical students, and allies, the society provides mentorship opportunities, regular educational seminars, research grants, and travel grants.[36] Other organizations, including *Nth Dimensions* and *The Perry Initiative,* work specifically to provide early exposure to orthopedic surgery for premedical and medical students. *Nth Dimensions* offers students from minoritized backgrounds a comprehensive, multi-pronged, strategic pipeline exposure to early clinical and research experience,[44] while *The Perry Initiative* offers 1-day hands-on programs to inspire women in high school, university, and medical school to pursue careers in orthopedic surgery and engineering.[37] The downstream effects of these organizations are remarkable. Research has found that women who attended *The Perry Initiative's Medical School Outreach Program* had a match rate of 20%, higher than the current percentage of women in orthopedic residencies,[46,47] and that the odds of applying into an orthopedic residency after *Nth Dimensions' Orthopedic Summer Internship Program* was 43.2 times higher among women and 14.5 times higher among underrepresented minorities.[21]

Newer initiatives include *Pride Ortho*, which aims to advance LGBTQ + representation in orthopedics through mentorship, educational resources, and scholarships,[43] as well as *#SpeakUpOrtho*, which provides a safe forum for orthopedic surgeons, fellows, attendings, and medical students to share experiences regarding microaggressions, bullying, harassment, and discrimination.[17,31] Finally, there are a number of more informal forums that bring together diverse groups, such as the *Women in Orthopedics* Facebook group with over 1800 members.

Professional Sports Initiative

To improve African American representation among *NFL* team physicians, the *National Football League Physicians Society* (*NFLPS*) and the *Professional Football*

Table 1
Summary of key diversity, equity, and inclusion organizations and initiatives in orthopedic surgery

Organization/Initiative		Target Population				Opportunities		
Name (hyperlinked)	Mission	High School/ Undergrad. Students	Medical Students	Residents/ Fellows	Attendings	Mentorship Programs	Educational Initiatives	Academic Grants/ Awards
Gender minorities								
Ruth Jackson Orthopedic Society[36]	To promote the professional development of women in orthopedics throughout all stages of their careers.	✔	✔	✔	✔	✔	✔	✔
The Perry Initiative[37]	To inspire young women to be leaders in the fields of orthopedic surgery and engineering by running hands-on outreach programs in high school, college, and medical school.	✔	✔			✔	✔	✔
Black Women Orthopedic Surgeons[38]	To support and empower Black women orthopedic surgeons through mentoring, activism, and education while advocating for health equity.		✔	✔	✔	✔	✔	
She Can Fix It Podcast[39]	To highlight and empower the women of orthopedic surgery.	✔	✔	✔	✔		✔	
Racial and ethnic minorities								
Black Women Orthopedic Surgeons[38]	As above							

(*continued on next page*)

Table 1
(continued)

Organization/Initiative		Target Population				Opportunities		
American Association of Latino Orthopedic Surgeons[40]	To promote the care of Latino patients by orthopedic surgeons and to promote greater diversity of professionals in the field.	✔	✔	✔	✔	✔	✔	✔
J. Robert Gladden Orthopedic Society[41,42]	To encourage, promote, and advance the science and medical art and practice of orthopedic surgery among African American, Black, and underrepresented minorities, as well as support orthopaedic-related studies of African American, Black, and underrepresented minority populations.	✔	✔	✔	✔	✔	✔	✔
Sexual minorities								
Pride Ortho[43]	To provide mentorship, networking, and belonging for lesbian, gay, bisexual, transgender, queer individuals, and allies in the orthopedic community.		✔	✔	✔	✔	✔	✔

Multiple minoritized identities								
Nth Dimensions[44]	To eliminate health care disparities in all communities by diversifying the physician workforce by implementing pipeline initiatives that provide resources and hands-on experience for women and underrepresented minorities.	✔	✔	✔		✔	✔	✔
International Orthopedic Diversity Alliance[45]	To champion diversity, equity, and inclusion in orthopedics worldwide.		✔	✔	✔	Developing	✔	Developing
Speak Up Ortho[31]	To increase awareness of bias, inequities, and harassment within orthopedic surgery.	✔	✔	✔	✔		✔	

Athletic Trainer Society launched an *NFL Diversity in Sports Medicine Pipeline Initiative* in 2022 to recruit medical students from 4 Historically Black Colleges and Universities to complete a clinical rotation with *NFL* club medical staff.[48] Medical students interested in sports medicine or orthopedic surgery from Charles R. Drew University of Medicine and Science, Howard University College of Medicine, Morehouse School of Medicine, and Meharry Medical College are selected by their respective schools to participate in a 1-month immersive clinical rotation with *NFL* medical staff. The goal of the program is to expose the student to the life and responsibilities of a team physician along with the full spectrum of training, rehabilitation, and therapeutic modalities that are integrated into the medical care of the players. A pilot program matching 2 students with 8 teams was completed by 16 students in the fall of 2022, all of whom returned to attend the *NFL Combine* in 2023. Building upon the successful pilot, the program is being expanded for anticipated participation by all 32 teams.

Stanford Initiatives

With successful orthopedic team physicians occupying the end of a long and rigorous pipeline, a comprehensive approach to enhancing diversity within the field of orthopedics is needed. Toward this goal, Stanford University School of Medicine and Stanford Orthopedic Surgery have implemented a multi-level and multi-year strategy focused on building a pipeline to support individuals from diverse backgrounds. As shown in **Fig. 3**, these initiatives begin as early as high school and continue through medical school, residency, fellowship, and into faculty recruitment and development.

High school

Stanford Orthopedics first partnered with *The Perry Initiative* (outlined above) in 2011 to offer yearly hands-on outreach programs for high school students interested in pursuing careers in orthopedic surgery and engineering. As part of these programs, students are able to participate in mock surgical exercises as well as attend lectures presented by female orthopedic surgeons and engineers at Stanford. Stanford offers these programs to foster an early interest in orthopedic surgery, reducing initial barriers to entry that may prevent women from pursuing this career. In 2022, 50 high school students attended the program, which is similar to the rates of attendance prior to the coronavirus disease 2019 pandemic.

University

At the university level, Stanford runs the *Racial Equity to Advance a Community of Health (REACH) Initiative* to train a generation of leaders in medicine and science to promote health equity, racial equity, and social justice. As part of this initiative, Stanford offers a *Post Baccalaureate Experience in Research* for underrepresented minorities and first-generation students. This program provides students with 1 to 2 years of rigorous research experience with Stanford faculty, tutoring for the Medical College Admission Test (MCAT), and guidance on medical school application preparation. Through this program, individuals who may not have otherwise had access to opportunities to succeed in the medical school application process will be able to prepare themselves to become competitive applicants. Additionally, Stanford offers its undergraduate students the opportunity to conduct research with orthopedic surgery faculty through accredited electives, thus exposing them early to the field.

Medical school

At the medical school level, Stanford has implemented several initiatives to ensure the success of each of its students, including MSK curricula, early clinical exposure, mentorship and research opportunities, and financial support.

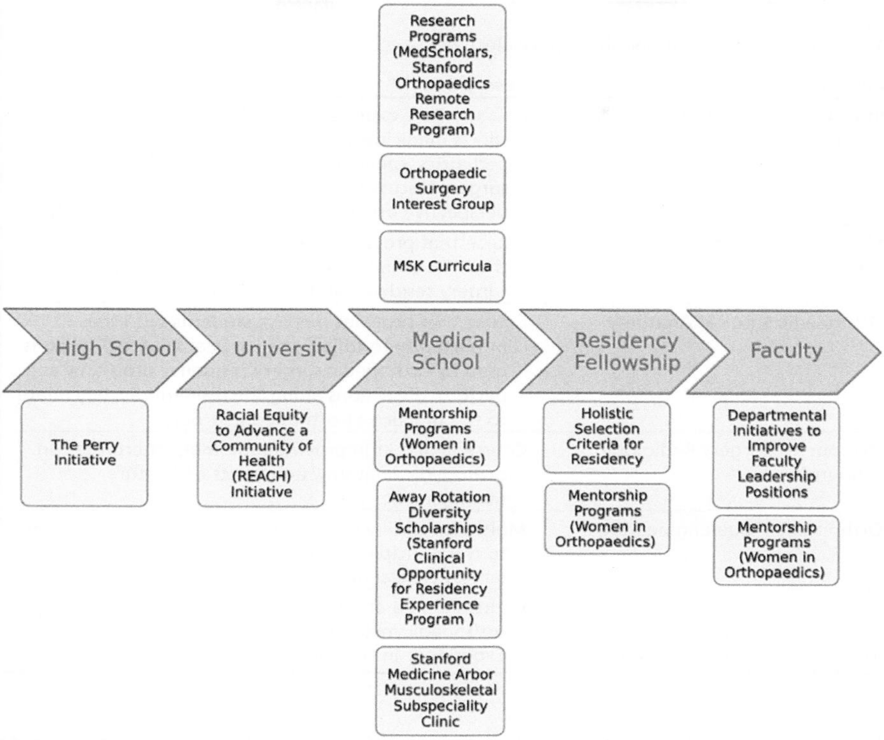

Fig. 3. Stanford University's pipeline approach to improving diversity in orthopedic surgery. Acronyms: Msk, musculoskeletal; REACH, racial equity to advance a community of health.

In addition to offering a mandatory MSK curriculum during the preclinical years, Stanford also offers a number of electives focused on orthopedic surgery. These electives, highlighted in **Table 2**, are intended to give students early exposure to orthopedic material as well as a means of establishing relationships with faculty and residents. Each year, students from diverse backgrounds enroll in the courses, offering early faculty exposure and chances to naturally find a mentor. Through the availability of these courses, all students have the equal opportunity to explore their potential interest in orthopedic surgery early in their medical careers, eliminating the common barrier that many students (especially those from diverse backgrounds) face in not being exposed to the field. Faculty at Stanford have also organized unique cadaveric dissection labs since 2015, wherein groups of medical students, residents, fellows, and faculty participate in 2-day intensive courses in Colorado, collecting data in order to improve understanding of pediatric knee development patterns and ligament reconstruction techniques.

In addition, the *Orthopedic Surgery Interest Group* (*OSIG*) holds free workshops for students on foundational orthopedic topics, and the *Stanford Medicine Arbor Musculoskeletal Subspeciality Clinic* provides students with the chance to provide free, culturally sensitive care to uninsured adults with MSK issues under the supervision of residents and attendings. Both the OSIG group as well as the specialty clinic have been increasingly led by women (2022–23: 75% and 100%, respectively; 2021–22: 50% and 50%, respectively), acting as a testimony to the growing female

Table 2
Stanford university orthopedic surgery electives

Course	Description
Introduction to Orthopedic Surgery	Course where experts from each subspecialty (including sports medicine, hand, shoulder, elbow, tumor, pediatrics, spine, and foot/ankle) in orthopedic surgery discuss their subspecialties and provide perspective on how to navigate them successfully.
Musculoskeletal (MSK) Examination Practicum	Course that provides practical, hands-on experience of the MSK examination facilitated by orthopedic surgery residents and attendings.
Orthopedic Surgical Anatomy	Course that provides medical students with the opportunity to follow the surgical anatomy syllabus used by orthopedic surgery residency programs and perform dissections alongside residents as they relate to the practice of orthopedic surgery.
Orthopedic Surgery Radiology Rounds	Course aimed at improving radiologic interpretation, orthopedic anatomy, and basics of fracture management.
Orthopedic Tissue Engineering	Multi-disciplinary course aimed at introducing students to the principles of tissue engineering through the lens of clinical need and translational research.
Early Clinical Experience in Orthopedic Surgery Introductory Clinical Mentorship	Courses aimed at pairing medical students with an orthopedic instructor to provide observational experience in the specialty.

interest in orthopedic surgery. Aside from providing students with opportunities to improve their clinical knowledge of orthopedic surgery, Stanford has implemented several mentorship and research programs. *Women in Orthopedics* is one of its mentorship programs, which offers an annual retreat for female medical students, residents, fellows, and faculty to network and foster mentorships. More than 20 mentorship pairings have formed via this initiative. Stanford also offers various research programs, including the *Medical Scholars Research Program* (*MedScholars*), which provides funding for Stanford medical students to conduct full-time research with a faculty mentor. In addition, Stanford aims to lower barriers for students from other institutions and underrepresented backgrounds to gain meaningful research and mentorship experiences through its *Stanford Orthopedics Remote Research Program*, a 10-week remote mentorship and clinical research program. During its pilot year in 2021, 17 students were selected to participate out of 115 applicants, and 9 faculty mentors were matched with 1 or 2 students.[49] Over the 3-month virtual curriculum, students conducted a research project with their assigned faculty member, as well as attended weekly lectures on research-related topics, orthopedic topics, diversity in medicine, leadership skills, and work-life balance.[49] This program was very successful in including participants from a diverse range of racial and ethnic backgrounds, geographic locations across the United States, and research experience levels, with a high rate of female participants (42%) and participants who identified as Black (35%).[49] Post-program surveys demonstrated that participants felt an improvement in their research skills and magnified their orthopedic interests.[49] This program has continued again in 2022 and 2023, with an increase in the number of applicants to 160 in 2022 and 270 in 2023, while continuing to successfully foster student and faculty mentorship with a focus on diversity, equity, and inclusion. Furthermore, Stanford

Medical School has Specialty Career Advisors for each medical sub-specialty, including an orthopedic surgery advisor, who is a woman.

In addition to supporting students during their pre-clerkship years, Stanford offers multiple clinical exposures to orthopedics through its home "clinical clerkship," home "clinical elective," and "sub-internship" offered to home and visiting students. Students also have the option of rotating on orthopedic services during their required core surgery rotation, giving them early exposure to the field prior to choosing electives. Furthermore, a 2-week or 4-week hand rotation is offered for those interested in this sub-specialty.

As a means of making sub-internship rotations as accessible as possible to visiting students, 2 programs for stipend support have been implemented. Since 2005, the Orthopedic Department Chair has written the Dean of Students at every allopathic medical school to notify them of stipend support for qualified sub-intern applicants who would potentially enhance the diversity of the Stanford orthopedic program. Stanford Medical School also developed the *Stanford Clinical Opportunity for Residency Experience Program (SCORE)*, which awards fourth-year medical students from diverse backgrounds a travel scholarship to support them during their away rotation as well as mentorship from Stanford faculty and residents with similar clinical interests.

Residency and fellowship

Extensive efforts have been made to improve the representation of residents through Stanford's implementation of a holistic selection process for interviewing and selecting residents. In addition to evaluating students' academic performances, Stanford considers their research experience, leadership positions, teamwork skills, and clinical performance during rotations. It has also created a goal of ensuring that the percentage of applicants from underrepresented backgrounds who are interviewed exceeds the percentage of applicants from underrepresented backgrounds who apply. Having acknowledged that research and leadership opportunities may not be equally distributed across academic institutions, Stanford Orthopedic Surgery has also developed and implemented programs to allow students from outside institutions to gain experience in these areas, such as through its remote research program discussed earlier.

Faculty

Stanford's departmental initiatives also aim to improve inclusivity and equity at the faculty level. Three of the five Vice Chairs appointed by the Department Chair are women. Of the 8 subspecialties in orthopedic surgery, 38% of the Division Chiefs are women, in juxtaposition with the national average of 9% (**Table 3**).[50] Additionally, the Chair of Santa Clara Valley Medical Center, which is affiliated with Stanford's orthopedic program, is a Hispanic woman. This is in a setting where the national average for female chairs is 3%.[50] At the faculty level, 1 in 5 attending surgeons is female. Many subspecialties exhibit substantial diversity, including foot/ankle surgery, hand/upper extremity surgery, and pediatric surgery. A diverse faculty at Stanford is important both for allowing students, residents, and fellows to see themselves in the field and for allowing patients from diverse backgrounds to receive care from providers who reflect their backgrounds.

Effect of pipeline initiatives

These pipeline initiatives have been successful. Over the last 10 years, the distribution of females rotating on clinical clerkships has nearly quadrupled, from around 9.7% in 2013 to 38% in 2023 (**Fig. 4**). There has also been a substantial increase in the representation of racial and ethnic minorities, with more than 50% of rotating students in the last year representing a racial or ethnic minority.

Table 3
Percentage of female orthopedic surgery chiefs and faculty at Stanford University

Orthopedic Subspeciality	Chief	% Female Faculty
Arthritis & Joint Replacement	Male	11% (1 in 9)
Foot & Ankle	Female	50% (2 in 4)
Hand & Upper Extremity	Female	38% (3 in 8)
MSK Tumor	Male	0% (0 in 3)
Orthopedic Trauma	Male	0% (0 in 4)
Pediatric Orthopedics	Male	33% (4 in 12)
Spine	Female	17% (1 in 6)
Sports Medicine	Male	8% (1 in 13)
Overall	38% (3 in 8)	21% (12 in 57[a])

[a] Total faculty number adds up to 59—2 removed because of joint appointments.

Each of the pipeline initiatives has been well received by students, encouraging them to participate in orthopedic care, research, and outreach. Ultimately, all the programs share a common theme—they seek to educate a diverse group of students interested in pursuing orthopedics and remove barriers that may prevent them from being able to do so.

In the past 4 years, over 40% of orthopedic surgery residents at Stanford University have been female, more than twice the national average (**Fig. 5**).[1] Stanford has also been ranked among the top 10 medical schools for producing the highest number of successful Black female applicants in orthopedic surgery.[51] It has not, however, ranked among the highest in terms of matching racial and ethnic minority residents into its residency program, highlighting an area for continued improvement.[51]

IMPLICATIONS/CONCLUSION

Although progress has been made to improve diversity in orthopedic surgery, the field as a whole still lags behind other medical and surgical specialties. Ensuring

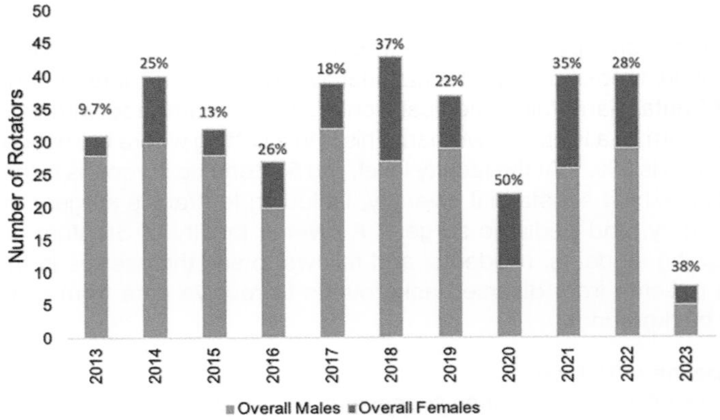

Fig. 4. Female representation in Stanford University orthopedic clerkships. Data include home and visiting students in Stanford's home clinical clerkship, home clinical elective, and sub-internship programs. Percentage above bars represents the female proportion. The year 2023 clerkships are underway.

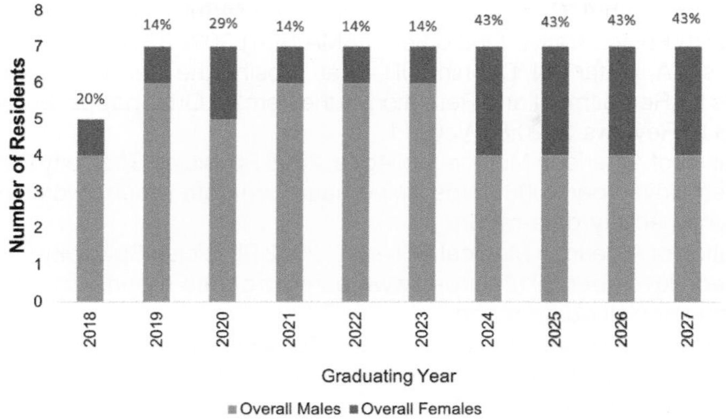

Fig. 5. Percentage of female orthopedic surgery residents at Stanford University in the past 10 years.

representation in orthopedic surgery and sports medicine is crucial for the success of programs and for the benefit of patients and athletes. To achieve this goal, orthopedic programs must implement pipeline initiatives to ensure that inclusivity is attained at all stages of professional development. Stanford University's pipeline approach to improving diversity in orthopedic surgery can serve as a model for other institutions. It involves providing early MSK didactic and clinical experiences; structured, longitudinal mentorship programs and research opportunities for students, residents, fellows, and attendings; and a demonstrated commitment to selecting, recruiting, and retaining individuals from a variety of backgrounds. In addition, there are numerous non-profit organizations actively engaged in orthopedic diversity initiatives outlined in this paper, which institutions and individuals can collaborate with. By acknowledging the importance of equity and inclusion and consciously implementing efforts to improve them, we can catalyze change in orthopedic surgery. Improving diversity in orthopedic surgery will provide the needed foundation for ensuring that more women and members of minority groups will serve as orthopedic team physicians at every level of sporting activity.

DISCLOSURE

The authors have no conflicts of interest to disclose.

REFERENCES

1. Day MA, Owens JM, Caldwell LS. Breaking Barriers: A Brief Overview of Diversity in Orthopedic Surgery. Iowa Orthop J 2019;39(1):1–5.
2. Association of American Medical Colleges. 2022 Physician Specialty Data Report. Published January 2023. https://www.aamc.org/data-reports/workforce/report/physician-specialty-data-report
3. Lamanna DL, Chen AF, Dyer GSM, et al. Diversity and Inclusion in Orthopaedic Surgery from Medical School to Practice: AOA Critical Issues. J Bone Joint Surg 2022;104(18):e80.
4. Wright MA, Murthi AM, Aleem A, et al. Patient Disparities and Provider Diversity in Orthopaedic Surgery: A Complex Relationship. J Am Acad Orthop Surg 2023;31(3):132–9.

5. Wallis CJD, Jerath A, Coburn N, et al. Association of Surgeon-Patient Sex Concordance With Postoperative Outcomes. JAMA Surg 2022;157(2):146.
6. Summers MA, Matar RN, Denning JR, et al. Closing the Gender Gap: Barriers to Success for Recruitment and Retention of the Female Orthopaedic Surgery Applicant. JBJS Reviews 2020;8(5):e0211.
7. Association of American Medical Colleges. 2008 Physician Specialty Data Report. Published November 2008. https://www.aamc.org/data-reports/workforce/report/physician-specialty-data-report
8. Association of American Medical Colleges. 2012 Physician Specialty Data Report. Published November 2012. https://www.aamc.org/data-reports/workforce/report/physician-specialty-data-report
9. Association of American Medical Colleges. 2014 Physician Specialty Data Report. Published November 2014. https://www.aamc.org/data-reports/workforce/report/physician-specialty-data-report
10. Association of American Medical Colleges. 2018 Physician Specialty Data Report. Published 2018. https://www.aamc.org/data-reports/workforce/report/physician-specialty-data-report
11. Association of American Medical Colleges. 2016 Physician Specialty Data Report. Published 2016. https://www.aamc.org/data-reports/workforce/report/physician-specialty-data-report
12. Association of American Medical Colleges. 2020 Physician Specialty Data Report. Published January 2021. https://www.aamc.org/data-reports/workforce/report/physician-specialty-data-report
13. Haffner MR, Van BW, Wick JB, et al. What is the Trend in Representation of Women and Under-represented Minorities in Orthopaedic Surgery Residency? Clin Orthop Relat Res 2021;479(12):2610–7.
14. National Resident Matching Program. National Resident Matching Program, Results and Data: 2021 Main Residency Match.; 2020.
15. National Resident Matching Program. National Resident Matching Program, Results and Data: 2021 Main Residency Match.; 2021.
16. National Resident Matching Program. National Resident Matching Program, Results and Data: 2022 Main Residency Match.; 2022.
17. Scerpella TA, Spiker AM, Lee CA, et al. Next Steps: Advocating for Women in Orthopaedic Surgery. J Am Acad Orthop Surg 2022;30(8):377–86.
18. Lin JS, Weber KL, Samora JB. How Does Representation of Women on Editorial Boards Compare Among Orthopaedic, General Surgery, and Internal Medicine Journals? Clin Orthop Relat Res 2021;479(9):1939–46.
19. Heest AV. Gender diversity in orthopedic surgery: We all know it's lacking, but why? Iowa Orthop J 2020;40(1):1–4.
20. Rahman R, Zhang B, Humbyrd CJ, et al. How Do Medical Students Perceive Diversity in Orthopaedic Surgery, and How Do Their Perceptions Change After an Orthopaedic Clinical Rotation? Clin Orthop Relat Res 2021;479(3):434–44.
21. Whicker E, Williams C, Kirchner G, et al. What Proportion of Women Orthopaedic Surgeons Report Having Been Sexually Harassed During Residency Training? A Survey Study. Clin Orthop Relat Res 2020;478(11):2598–606.
22. Balch Samora J, Van Heest A, Weber K, et al. Harassment, Discrimination, and Bullying in Orthopaedics: A Work Environment and Culture Survey. J Am Acad Orthop Surg 2020;28(24):e1097–104.
23. Okike K, Phillips DP, Swart E, et al. Orthopaedic Faculty and Resident Sex Diversity Are Associated with the Orthopaedic Residency Application Rate of Female Medical Students. J Bone Joint Surg 2019;101(12):e56.

24. Rohde RS, Wolf JM, Adams JE. Where Are the Women in Orthopaedic Surgery? Clin Orthop Relat Res 2016;474(9):1950–6.
25. Johnson AL, Sharma J, Chinchilli VM, et al. Why Do Medical Students Choose Orthopaedics as a Career? J Bone Joint Surg 2012;94(11):e78.
26. London DA, Calfee RP, Boyer MI. Impact of a Musculoskeletal Clerkship on Orthopedic Surgery Applicant Diversity. Am J Orthop (Belle Mead NJ) 2016; 45(6):E347–51.
27. McDonald TC, Drake LC, Replogle WH, et al. Barriers to Increasing Diversity in Orthopaedics. JB JS Open Access 2020;5(2):e0007.
28. Hill JF, Yule A, Zurakowski D, et al. Residents' Perceptions of Sex Diversity in Orthopaedic Surgery. J Bone Joint Surg 2013;95(19):e144.
29. Malige A, Wells L, Brooks JT, et al. A Cross-Sectional Evaluation of the Successful Minority Applicant to Orthopaedic Surgery Residency Programs. J Racial Ethn Health Disparities 2022;9(6):2164–70.
30. Samora JB, Denning J, Haralabatos S, et al. Do women experience microaggressions in orthopaedic surgery? Current state and future directions from a survey of women orthopaedists. Current Orthopaedic Practice 2020;31(5):503–7.
31. Gianakos AL, Mulcahey MK, Weiss JM, et al. SpeakUpOrtho: Narratives of Women in Orthopaedic Surgery—Invited Manuscript. J Am Acad Orthop Surg 2022;30(8):369–76.
32. Bohl DD, Iantorno SE, Kogan M. Inappropriate Questions Asked of Female Orthopaedic Surgery Applicants From 1971 to 2015: A Cross-sectional Study. J Am Acad Orthop Surg 2019;27(14):519–26.
33. O'Connor MI. Medical School Experiences Shape Women Students' Interest in Orthopaedic Surgery. Clin Orthop Relat Res 2016;474(9):1967–72.
34. Burton É, Flores B, Jerome B, et al. Assessment of Bias in Patient Safety Reporting Systems Categorized by Physician Gender, Race and Ethnicity, and Faculty Rank: A Qualitative Study. JAMA Netw Open 2022;5(5):e2213234.
35. Ode GE, Brooks JT, Middleton KK, et al. Perception of Racial and Intersectional Discrimination in the Workplace Is High Among Black Orthopaedic Surgeons: Results of a Survey of 274 Black Orthopaedic Surgeons in Practice. J Am Acad Orthop Surg 2022;30(1):7–18.
36. Ruth Jackson, Orthopaedic Society. Ruth Jackson Orthopaedic Society. Published 2023. http://www.rjos.org/
37. The Perry Initiative. The Perry Initiative. Published 2023. https://perryinitiative.org/
38. Black Women Orthopaedic Surgeons. Black Women Orthopaedic Surgeons. Published 2023. https://bwos.org/
39. She Can Fix It Podcast. She Can Fix It Podcast. Published 2023. https://www.shecanfixitpod.com/
40. American Association of Latino Orthopaedic Surgeons. American Association of Latino Orthopaedic Surgeons. Published 2023. https://www.aalos.org/
41. J. Robert Gladden Orthopaedic Society. J. Robert Gladden Orthopaedic Society. Published 2023. https://www.gladdensociety.org/
42. Brooks JT, Taylor E, Peterson D, et al. The J. Robert Gladden Orthopaedic Society: Past, Present, and Future. J Am Acad Orthop Surg 2021;17. https://doi.org/10.5435/JAAOS-D-21-01129.
43. Pride Ortho. Pride Ortho. Published 2023. https://prideortho.org/
44. Nth Dimensions. Nth Dimensions. Published 2023. https://www.nthdimensions.org/
45. International Orthopaedic Diversity Alliance. International Orthopaedic Diversity Alliance. Published 2023. https://www.orthopaedicdiversity.org/

46. Harbold D, Dearolf L, Buckley J, et al. The Perry Initiative's Impact on Gender Diversity Within Orthopedic Education. Curr Rev Musculoskelet Med 2021;14(6): 429–33. https://doi.org/10.1007/s12178-021-09717-4.
47. Mason BS, Ross W, Ortega G, et al. Can a Strategic Pipeline Initiative Increase the Number of Women and Underrepresented Minorities in Orthopaedic Surgery? Clin Orthop Relat Res 2016;474(9):1979–85. https://doi.org/10.1007/s11999-016-4846-8.
48. Grant M, Weiss A, Weir L. NFL Launches Initiative to Increase Diversity in Sports Medicine. NFL.com. Published May 24, 2022. https://www.nfl.com/playerhealthandsafety/resources/press-releases/nfl-launches-initiative-to-increase-diversity-in-sports-medicine
49. Hastings KG, Freiman HD, Amanatullah DF, et al. A Pilot Program: Remote Summer Program to Improve Opportunity and Mentorship Among Underrepresented Students Pursuing Orthopaedic Surgery. JB JS Open Access 2022;7(4): e2200059. https://doi.org/10.2106/JBJS.OA.22.00059.
50. Bi AS, Fisher ND, Bletnitsky N, et al. Representation of Women in Academic Orthopaedic Leadership: Where Are We Now? Clin Orthop Relat Res 2022;480(1): 45–56. https://doi.org/10.1097/CORR.0000000000001897.
51. Nsekpong TB, Ode G, Purcell K, et al. A track record of diversity: Medical schools ranked by successful black applicants to orthopaedic residencies. Journal of the National Medical Association 2022;114(2):156–66. https://doi.org/10.1016/j.jnma.2021.12.013.

Efforts to Improve Diversity, Equality, and Inclusion in Sports Medicine via Community Engagement Initiatives Within American Cities Divided by Racial, Social, and Economic Factors

Michael D. Maloney, MD[a,b,*], Ram Haddas, PhD[a,b], Edward M. Schwarz, PhD[a,b], Shaun Nelms, EdD[a,b], Katherine Rizzone, MD[a,b]

KEYWORDS

• Disparities • Injury prevention • Physical activity intervention • Wearables

KEY POINTS

- The huge disparities in socioeconomics, education, and health between teens living in urban poverty and under-resourced school districts versus adequately resourced teens must be understood and respected before attempting an athletic performance and injury prevention program with this underserved demographic.
- Although the structure, goals, and primary outcomes of disparate urban versus middle class suburban athletic performance and injury prevention programs for youth differ, both populations need these interventions.
- Pilot data exist demonstrating the feasibility of an orthopedic department-based community engagement initiative for evidence-based athletic performance and injury prevention programs in both disparate urban and middle class suburban high schools with potential enhancement by online and wearable device technologies.

Central motivations for this text, *Equality, Diversity, and Inclusion in Sports Medicine*, are the well-established disparities between economically challenged underperforming school districts and geographically adjacent middle class suburban schools and the male versus female athletic programs within these schools throughout the United

[a] Center for Musculoskeletal Research, University of Rochester Medical Center, Rochester, NY, USA; [b] Department of Orthopedics and Rehabilitation, University of Rochester Medical Center, Rochester, NY, USA
* Corresponding author. Department of Orthopaedics, Stromg Memorial Hospital, 601 Elmwood Avenue, Box 665, Rochester, NY 14642.
E-mail address: mike_maloney@urmc.rochester.edu

Clin Sports Med 43 (2024) 271–277
https://doi.org/10.1016/j.csm.2023.06.010

States. Thus, this article assumes that the reader is generally familiar with these facts and that the need for community outreach programs to address these problems is both self-evident and exceedingly challenging due to social, political, and economic factors that thwart most well-intentioned interventions. As we are very far from prescriptive community outreach programs with proven outcomes and it is acknowledged that every community is different such that successful interventions must be tailored, here we merely describe the experience of the Center for Human Athleticism, Musculoskeletal Performance and Prevention (CHAMPP) pilot program at the University of Rochester as a contemporary example of an academic Orthopedic Department's efforts to address these problems.

ROCHESTER, NY: A TYPICAL US CITY IN DECLINE WITH MAJOR DISPARITY ISSUES

With a population of ~200,000 residents, Rochester is the fourth largest city in New York state based on the 2020 US census and is surrounded by ~1 million people in neighboring suburban and rural communities within the Finger Lakes Region of the state. The Seneca Nation of Native Americans lived in and around Rochester before losing claim of the land in the Treaty of Big Tree in 1797, and the city's origins commenced with the land purchased by Colonel Nathaniel Rochester in 1803, for whom the city is named. From a population and economic standpoint, Rochester achieved its peak in the 1950s to 1960s, largely due to its industrial corporate giants, Eastman Kodak, Xerox, and Bausch & Lomb, whose subsequent demise left the city in financial ruin. Concurrent with this downturn, institutional racism (ie, redlining), and the development of food deserts, the city's demographics changed from being predominantly White upper and middle class, to its current population that is 37% Black or African American (Non-Hispanic), 15% Hispanic, and 36% White (Non-Hispanic). Perhaps the most tragic consequence has been the fate of Rochester's urban children, most of whom live in poverty which the US Census Bureau defines as a family of four making less than $27,750 a year and attend Rochester Central School District (RCSD) high schools that have a twenty-first-century graduation rate of ~40%. In stark contrast, children who live in the adjunct suburbs in Monroe County, which is 74% White, 10% Black or African American (Non-Hispanic), and 8% Hispanic, attend public high schools with ~95% graduation rates and several have been ranked within the top 100 in the United States.

Equally important to the background of the CHAMPP pilot is an understanding of the University of Rochester Medical Center (URMC), which has an annual budget of $3.8 billion, is wholly owned by the private University, and is located within the city of Rochester. In addition to its urban main campus, UR Medicine is Upstate New York's largest and most comprehensive health care system, with more than 26,000 employees, staffs six other hospitals, and many outpatient facilities throughout the region. This makes the University of Rochester the largest private sector employer based in Upstate New York and the sixth-largest employer in the state.

With this background, the following summary of the CHAMPP pilot and its future directions were written with four theses in mind: (1) Rochester, NY is not atypical of most US boomtowns that achieved population and wealth peaks as large cities during America's industrial period and now suffer from economic downturn that contributes to racial disparities in health and wellness. (2) The macroeconomics and wellness of these American cities are now significantly controlled by very large health care systems, as National Health Expenditures now account for 20% of the Gross Domestic Product, and the embedded academic medical institution within bears a fiduciary role in developing community outreach interventions to address disparities, which also benefit the health care system. (3) Inequities exist in both financially challenged underperforming urban high schools and their neighboring upper- and middle-class high schools, but outreach programs to address them must understand these distinct communities and run interventions accordingly. (4) Fitness Science interventions can be implemented to improve high school student personal wellness, accountability and healthy lifestyle decision making in both communities.

The Center for Human Athleticism, Musculoskeletal Performance and Prevention

The origins of the CHAMPP pilot commenced around 2008 with the national rage about childhood obesity, teen suicide, and the high rate of serious sport injuries in female high school athletes. At this time, the Sports Medicine Division of the Department of Orthopedics at URMC had five attending surgeons who scheduled physician coverage of greater than 20 Rochester suburban high school football games as well as provided access for acute injuries within 24 hours and a separate Saturday afternoon sports injury clinic focused on local college and high school athletes. Through this interaction and by observing various deficiencies in athletic training for competitive varsity high school sports, the opportunity presented to propose a fee-for-service program to the athletic directors of the suburban high schools. These community outreach programs, now referred to as CHAMPP Retail, involve URMC Athletic Training and Performance staff, who run Fitness Science clinics in the suburban high school gyms 2 or 3 days per week. Currently, there are greater than 25 CHAMPP Retail programs in Rochester, and we are beginning to quantify their outcomes and cost-effectiveness. Importantly, the successful revenue stream from CHAMPP Retail allowed us to explore non-fee-for-service programs with disadvantaged Rochester youth. Unfortunately, due to major financial, liability, and distrust issues, URMC Sports Medicine was denied access to athletes at all RCSD school until 2018.

University of Rochester Educational Partnership Organization for East High School and Center for Human Athleticism, Musculoskeletal Performance and Prevention Urban

Of the RCSD high schools, East High School (EHS) was one of the worst academic performers and failed to meet most New York state benchmarks in the 1990s and 2000s. East, the district's oldest, largest school, served grades 7 to 12, with students organized into a lower school (grades 7–8) and an upper school (9–12). Within its student body, 54% of scholars identify as Black, 34% Latinx, 8% white, 3% Asian, and 1% multiracial, and 86% qualify as economically disadvantaged. At the time, the partnership began, only 33% of East's seniors graduated on time, the dropout rate was 41%, there were 2468 annual suspensions, and attendance was 77%. This triggered the New York State Education Department (NYSED) to mandate its closure, pending approval of an Educational Partnership Organization (EPO, legal equivalent to superintendent) to oversee all employees and activities on a daily basis. In April 2014, the University of Rochester agreed to the request by the RCSD Board of Education to become the EPO for EHS, which was approved by NYSED for the 2015 to 2016 school year.[1] These decisions and subsequent actions have been transformative for all involved,[1] most notably the children of Rochester, and those interested in learning more about the truly incredible reversal in all metrics of behavior (ie, incarcerations, teen pregnancies, expulsions, suspensions) and academics (ie, grade point average, graduation rate, enrollment in high education) are encouraged to search the Internet as a formal literature has yet to be published.

Before 2018, gaining access to scholars and families within the RCSD was difficult due to RCSDs constant change in leadership and lack of organizational coherence.

The EPO university–school partnership provided an opportunity for CHAMPP to gain access to scholars, families, and resources within the RCSD without unnecessary delays.[2] With EPO access to RCSD high school students, gym space donated by the Penfield Young Men's Christian Association (YMCA) partially in response to four teen suicides within 16 months in its small suburban community, and food donated by Wegmans Inc, URMC Sports Medicine undertook a bold and novel Fitness Science community outreach pilot program in the fall of 2018 in which it combined high performing varsity athletes in the CHAMPP Retail program at Webster high school (White male and female children, $n = 15$), with varsity athletes at EHS (Black male and female children, $n = 15$).[3] This program was free to all participants, and the staffing and EHS student transportation were funded by URMC. As the sustainability of this non-fee-for-service pilot program, termed CHAMPP Urban, was dependent on quantitative return on investment (ROI), the directors of the program incorporated UR and RCSD institutional review board (IRB)-approved human subjects research protocols to assess the efficacy of a 10-week Fitness Science program using Patient-Reported Outcomes Measurement Information System (PROMIS) and Functional Movement Screening (FMS) as the primary outcome measures.[3] No adverse events of the training or study were reported, and Kaplan–Meier assessment demonstrated excellent retention throughout the 10 weeks. Although no effects on fatigue and physical function were found, suggesting that greater than 10-week is required, the intervention significantly improved anxiety, peer relationships, pain interference, and trended toward significance for depression ($P < .05$).[3] Also of note, bench press, combined Pro Agility, and total FMS were all significantly improved ($P < .05$). Remarkably, there were 10 students (67%) in peril of sports-related injury (FM < 14) at the start of the intervention, and all but one (90%) eliminated this serious risk factor. Most importantly, these data published in the peer-reviewed literature[3] provided CHAMPP Urban the ROI it needed to gain sustained support from EHS coaches and students, URMC, and local philanthropy to establish a long-term Fitness Science program for disadvantaged Rochester youth.

Use of Wearable Devices to Enhance Participation and Outcomes

The 2018 pilot also demonstrates the feasibility of PROMIS and FMS outcomes, which enabled competitive public and private grant funding to improve and expand CHAMPP Urban. An example was a subsequent IRB-approved human subject study of RCSD students, which was funded by grants from the National Institutes of Health and the Konar Foundation and assessed the feasibility of using wearables (Fitbit) to evaluate the effects of Fitness Science training on the daily activity of minority female athletes at EHS.[4] Of note is that a motivation for this research study was the frank obesity and lack of self-reported sleep in the first EHS cohort, begging an automated reporting system within the intervention to constantly monitor vigorous activity and rapid eye movement sleep. We also aimed to identify candidate Fitbit outcome measures for future prospective CHAMPP Retail and CHAMPP Urban studies. Five out of twenty-four RCSD female students in the 10-week CHAMPP Urban pilot were provided Fitbit devices, from which we obtained data sets from three students. The data showed that although compliance was challenging, wearable devices could be used to evaluate daily physical activity (PA) levels and intensities in underrepresented minority high school female athletes during an extended PA intervention.[4] We also found that the assessment of moderate-vigorous activity (min/d) was the best measure of global PA using Fitbit.[4] As these wearable devices provided freely to participates have ROI and are viewed as incentives for both urban and suburban students, we recommend them in all Fitness Science community outreach interventions.

With these promising results using wearables to assess functional outcome measurements (FOMs) in under-representative populations along with the advancement of wearables technology in health care and sports medicine, wearables play a vital role in the success of the CHAMPP program. The term wearable refers to a wide range of small, noninvasive integrated computing devices that can be worn by a person. The application of wearable technology in sports medicine comes in different forms and can differ based on its application and the goals of the user. The popular ones are body-worn devices (wrist), but there are other types, such as sensor-embedded equipment and smart textiles.[5,6] Common places for sensors are performance-based and may be located in the insole, helmet, pad, and tactical vest.[5–7] Wearables consumers are often driven by the opportunity to improve performance, gaining valuable data from tracking personal functions (eg, Fitbit, daily step tracking, or caloric utilization).[6,8] Wearable devices are capable of collecting continuous sensor data over the course of days, weeks, and months. This can provide a longitudinal representation of the general health and mobility of the wearer, as opposed to the time-dependent and subjective PROMIS and in-office physical assessment.[9] By collecting FOMs accurately through wearables, we will be able to corroborate these with PROMIS, as we have already done with CHAMPP program.

STEP at the YMCA

Disparities in sports participation and PA occur at a young age and are often intersectional.[10] Demographics such as gender, race, ethnicity, disability,[11] sexual orientation,[12] gender identity,[12] primary language, and geography[13] are all factors in how active an individual is, because they impact the opportunities offered.[14] Social determinants of health (SDOH) are an additional layer that impacts individuals' access to sports and exercise.[15] Examples of SDOH that can impact sports participation and PA levels include transportation security, grocery store location, and neighborhood safety.[16]

The recommended PA guidelines for adolescents are 60 minutes of moderate PA 7 days a week with at least 3 days a week involving vigorous activity. According to NHANES data, 47.8% of adolescents do not meet any part of this recommendation and less than 20% meet the full guidelines. Even more concerning is the gender and racial disparity that exists within these numbers, particularly females of color, who have lower levels of PA compared with other demographic groups. This discrepancy begins early in life, commencing in adolescence. Once a lifestyle of physical inactivity has been established, it can be difficult to make meaningful behavior change later in life, which has significant ramifications, as these populations are at greater risk for the development of cardiovascular disease and other comorbidities compared with their white and male counterparts. Increasing PA in young females during the formative time of adolescence may lead to positive lifelong effects in health and wellness and may help prevent cardiovascular comorbidities.

Multiple interventions have been created, implemented, and evaluated in inactive, adolescent populations, but few of them have been designed with input from potential participants, and many do not lead to a long-term increase in PA. In our community-based program, we attempted to take these factors into consideration. Before designing our activity intervention, we conducted the focus groups of adolescents, parents, educators, and community members to explore barriers and facilitators of PA among Black and Brown women in the city of Rochester. We identified motivators for exercise and activity and also gathered suggestions from our participants about the potential design of our program, allowing them to take the lead. Using these data, we created a participant-driven intervention Student Teacher Exercise Program (STEP) at the inner city YMCA that was based in increasing PA while also incorporating other aspects to address barriers to activity we heard in the focus groups.

One of the key points taken from our experience in working in the community is that COVID-19 negatively impacted sports participation and PA in this community. Urban schools have larger proportions of students of color. Urban schools were more often to be virtually based during the pandemic, making it more difficult for student athletes to participate in their sports. It also made it more difficult for nonathletes to be active as well because PA classes were also virtual. Aspects to consider are that some students enjoyed this type of engagement, doing more social media challenges versus in-person classes and may have been more inclusive to those students with disabilities. Although the pandemic has offered the opportunity to be engaged with students and student athletes in novel ways, in general students who were a member of a marginalized community were more likely to be less active during the pandemic.

FUTURE DIRECTIONS

The authors are encouraged and motivated by the acceptance of the CHAMPP program by not only the students at EHS but also the teachers and administrators. This ongoing collaboration provides a tremendous opportunity to engage more participants. We also are hopeful of scaling our program to other schools across RCSD. The successes mentioned above have gained the interest of additional philanthropic support as well as the attention of city and state educators. However, peer-reviewed publications on the outcomes and cost-effectiveness of the pilots are needed for broad adoption and sustainable funding.

We also see wearable devices as an integral part of CHAMPP. Theses wearable devices could help us, educators and clinicians, engage students more deeply. To a student, these devices could be a way to stay connected to their clinicians and educators and make them feel more involved in their care. The longitudinal aspect of these wearable devices will hopefully improve the clinicians–student relationship. By combining wearables with artificial intelligence, wearable devices could be used in the future to create predictive algorithms and diagnose diseases.[9] Moreover, students can benefit from wearable sensors by receiving biofeedback and reducing mechanical risk factors by implementing these measurements in their daily lives. As well as supporting user monitoring, they could facilitate and encourage self-management among students.[17] Understanding these devices' data, addressing students' concerns about the privacy of these data, and improving preventative care are critical for clinicians and educators.

DISCLOSURE

The authors have no conflicts of interest to disclose.

GRANT FUNDING

This work was supported by grants from the Konar Foundation and the National Institutes of Health, United States (P30 AR069655).

REFERENCES

1. Larson J, Nelms S. Collaborating for Equity in Urban Education: Comprehensive Reform in an Innovative University/School Partnership. Urban Educ 2021;0. https://doi.org/10.1177/00420859211017976.
2. Marsh VL, Nelms SC, Peyre S, et al. How a university and a school district made change together. Phi Delta Kappan 2022;104(2):37–43.

3. Cole CL, Vasalos K, Nicandri G, et al. Use of PROMIS and Functional Movement System (FMS) Testing to Evaluate the Effects of Athletic Performance and Injury Prevention Training in Female High School Athletes. Orthop Sports Med 2019; 3(2):255–8. Epub 2020/02/11.
4. Cole CL, Vasalos K, Nicandri G, et al. Use of Fitbit Data to Evaluate the Effects of an Athletic Performance and Injury Prevention Training Program on Daily Physical Levels in Underrepresented Minority Female High School Athletes: A Prospective Study. Orthop Sports Med 2020;4(2):370–6. Epub 2020/11/10.
5. Kamisalic A, Fister I Jr, Turkanovic M, et al. Sensors and Functionalities of Non-Invasive Wrist-Wearable Devices: A Review. Sensors 2018;18(6). Epub 20180525.
6. Aroganam G, Manivannan N, Harrison D. Review on Wearable Technology Sensors Used in Consumer Sport Applications. Sensors 2019;19(9). Epub 20190428.
7. Johnston W, Heiderscheit B, Coughlan G, et al. Concussion Recovery Evaluation Using the Inertial Sensor Instrumented Y Balance Test. J Neurotrauma 2020; 37(23):2549–57. Epub 20200708.
8. Lee TJ, Galetta MS, Nicholson KJ, et al. Wearable Technology in Spine Surgery. Clin Spine Surg 2020 Jul;33(6):218–21.
9. Mobbs RJ, Fonseka RD, Natarajan P. Wearable sensor technology in spine care. J Spine Surg 2022;8(1):84–6.
10. Whitt-Glover MC, Taylor WC, Floyd MF, et al. Disparities in physical activity and sedentary behaviors among US children and adolescents: prevalence, correlates, and intervention implications. J Publ Health Pol 2009;30(1):S309–34.
11. Ross SM, Smit E, Yun J, et al. Updated national estimates of disparities in physical activity and sports participation experienced by children and adolescents with disabilities: NSCH 2016–2017. J Phys Activ Health 2020;17(4):443–55.
12. Calzo JP, Roberts AL, Corliss HL, et al. Physical activity disparities in heterosexual and sexual minority youth ages 12–22 years old: roles of childhood gender nonconformity and athletic self-esteem. Annals of behavioral medicine 2014; 47(1):17–27.
13. Kenney MK, Wang J, Iannotti R. Residency and racial/ethnic differences in weight status and lifestyle behaviors among US youth. J Rural Health 2014;30(1): 89–100.
14. Gortmaker SL, Lee R, Cradock AL, et al. Disparities in youth physical activity in the United States: 2003-2006. Med Sci Sports Exerc 2012;44(5):888–93.
15. Marmot M, Allen JJ. Social determinants of health equity. American Public Health Association; 2014. p. S517–9.
16. Social Determinants of Health. U.S. Department of Health and Human Services 2022 cited 2022; Available from: https://health.gov/healthypeople/priority-areas/social-determinants-health.
17. Triantafyllou A, Papagiannis G, Stasi S, et al. Application of Wearable Sensors Technology for Lumbar Spine Kinematic Measurements during Daily Activities following Microdiscectomy Due to Severe Sciatica. Biology 2022;11(3). Epub 20220303.

Sports Medicine Patient Experience: Implicit Bias Mitigation and Communication Strategies

Pedro J. Tort Saadé, MD[a,b,*], Augustus A. White III, MD-PhD[c]

KEYWORDS

• Sports medicine • Athletes • Communication strategies • Implicit bias • Mitigation • Equality • Diversity • Inclusion

KEY POINTS

- Implicit biases are developed over a lifetime through people's experiences, eventually influencing postures towards multiple choices like race, ethnicity, and physical appearance.
- Education and self-awareness about implicit bias and its potentially harmful effects on judgment and behavior may lead individuals to pursue corrective action and mitigation.
- Team physicians must consider race, gender, critical social determinants of health, access to care, and patient expectations, all of which can significantly impact patient outcomes.
- The first step in preventing implicit bias is educating ourselves about the spontaneous cognitive processes that unconsciously affect our clinical decisions.

INTRODUCTION

In the last decade, many organizations have been working toward achieving equitable and unbiased interaction and opportunities for all types of people. However, persistent racial inequalities and attitudes have driven a search for factors generating ongoing discrimination. Multiple investigators have inculpated implicit race biases as the principal contributor to the perpetuation of discrimination.[1–4] Unconscious bias occurs spontaneously and unintentionally, affecting the judgment, decision-making, outcomes, and athlete's care.[1,5] Therefore, education and self-awareness about implicit bias are paramount to swift

[a] Surgery Department, Doctors' Center Hospital San Juan, San Juan, Puerto Rico; [b] Universidad Central del Caribe School of Medicine, Bayamon, Puerto Rico; [c] Ellen and Melvin Gordon Distinguished Professor Emeritus of Medical Education and Professor Emeritus of Orthopedic Surgery at Harvard Medical School, Boston, MA, USA
* Corresponding author. Pmb 318, 138 Winston Churchill Avenue, San Juan, PR 00926-6023.
E-mail address: ptortsaade@gmail.com

Clin Sports Med 43 (2024) 279–291
https://doi.org/10.1016/j.csm.2023.07.002
0278-5919/24/

individuals to pursue corrective actions and mitigation strategies to improve team physician-athlete relationships, athlete's performance, well-being, and care.[6]

HISTORY

The term "implicit bias" was portrayed in 1995 by psychologists Mahzarin Banaji and Anthony Greenwald[7] as a social behavior primarily influenced by unconscious associations and judgments. After further author contributions, the term was defined as "the unconscious stereotyping and formation of attitudes toward groups or ideas that can influence our actions." For example, individuals may fully support equality, but their cognition could unknowingly persuade them to react differently.[8]

The concept of implicit bias was initially theorized in 2013 by authors Mahzarin Banaji and Anthony Greenwald in a book called "Blindspot: Hidden Biases of Good People." They explored humans' hidden biases due to life experiences and factors such as nationality, age, gender, ethnicity, and religion. "Humans possess mental blindspots like our visual blind spots—they exist without conscious awareness." "These blindspots house our hidden biases, or 'mind bugs,' which directly conflict with our conscious beliefs and ideologies."[6]

The hidden biases concept is based on prevailing ideas in psychology that the unconscious mind is responsible for much of our actions and behavior. Therefore, humans possess unconscious biases that contribute to discrimination. The mind has an automatic or unconscious side and the reflective or conscious side. Hidden biases are a by-product of the unconscious side and may interfere with the actions and behaviors of the reflective and conscious side.[6]

DEFINITIONS

Implicit bias is a form of bias that occurs spontaneously and unintentionally and nevertheless affects judgments, decisions, and behaviors. It is also known as unconscious bias, is often automatically activated, and operates at a level below the consciousness.[1] It is an unconscious preference in judgment and behavior that results from subtle cognitive processes.[9]

Implicit bias is usually built up based on implicit attitudes and stereotypes, is not limited to race, and can exist for attributes including gender, age, gender identity, disability status, sexual orientation, and physical characteristics such as color, height, and weight. The stereotypes about people are practically ubiquitous, and the implicit bias occurs automatically in almost everyone. Implicit biases are developed over a lifetime through people's environments and experiences. They will eventually influence feelings and attitudes toward multiple choices such as race, ethnicity, physical appearance, and age.[9]

BACKGROUND

Implicit biases are linked to prejudiced outcomes such as poorer quality interactions,[10] constrained employment opportunities,[11] and a decreased probability of receiving life-saving emergency medical care.[6] Moreover, many theorists concluded that implicit biases persist and are robust determinants of behavior because people lack personal awareness of them. They can happen despite conscious nonprejudiced intentions.[1,4,12]

Unconscious bias can influence the patient-provider relationship, treatment decisions, and outcomes. A systematic review by Hall and colleagues found that implicit bias was significantly related to patient-provider interactions, treatment decisions, treatment adherence, and patient health outcomes.[5] The group concluded that

"Implicit attitudes were more often significantly related to patient-provider interactions and health outcomes than treatment processes."

Unconscious bias is an implicit bias that can be considered a "*shortcut*" our minds take to make a rapid and spontaneous judgment about someone.[13,14] Personal background, life experiences, societal stereotypes, and cultural background influence perceptions and decisions about interactions with others. The associations are based on multiple experiences and direct and indirect exposures during life, starting at a very early age.

Differences in gender, ethnicity, race, and socioeconomic status within the diverse population of the United States have led to the infiltration of disparities across many specialties in the medical field.[15,16] Several investigators have documented differences in orthopedics utilization, selection, treatment, and outcomes.[15,17–21] In 2003, in the Institute of Medicine report "Unequal Treatment: Confronting Racial and Ethnic Disparities in Health Care," the investigators determined that "bias, stereotyping, and clinical uncertainty on the part of health care providers may contribute to racial and ethnic disparities in health care" often despite providers' best intentions.[22]

Several studies have shown that individual and institutional discrimination contributes to disparities in African American patients, resulting in fewer indicated and required procedures and higher infant mortality rates compared with non-Hispanic whites.[22,23]

Female athletes are 2 to 8 times more likely to sustain an anterior cruciate ligament (ACL) injury.[23–25] Hence, recent literature on ACL injuries in women has shown an interest in understanding the potential mechanism underlying gender differences in injury rates.[26] In addition, several investigators have documented multifactorial reasons for racial and ethnic disparities in treatment and outcomes after ACL injuries in the population.[27] Furthermore, patient satisfaction and health outcomes are favorable when racial, ethnic, and linguistic concordance exists between the physician and patient.[28–30]

In recent years, multiple reports in the literature have documented the concept that implicit bias in health care can directly lead to health care disparities. Eliminating health care disparities is among the top 5 initiatives of the National Institute of Health. The concept of implicit bias mitigations in health adopts multiple strategies to identify and make people aware of each person's elements for judgment and how to avoid unconscious bias and improve behavior, health care–patient interactions, and outcomes. Burgess and colleagues documented that "if health care providers understand that stereotyping and racial prejudice are 'a normal aspect of human cognition,' they may be more open to learning about this phenomenon and how it impacts medical practice."[31]

Druckman and colleagues did a study and evaluated race and sports and focused on racial bias in the sports medicine field. The investigators evaluated the interaction of racial bias in pain-related perceptions among NCAA Division I sports medical staff. The study results showed that medical staff perceived black athletes as feeling less pain than white counterparts and basketball players as feeling less pain than soccer players. Moreover, the bias was mediated by perceptions of social class. Racial bias was not evident in other outcome measures, including the perception of recovery process pain, the likelihood of overreporting pain, and the overuse of drugs to combat pain.[32]

Devana and colleagues[27] conducted a research study to review the literature to identify gender, racial and ethnic disparities in incidence, treatment, and outcomes of ACL injury. The study results showed that non-White and Spanish-speaking patients are less likely to undergo anterior cruciate ligament reconstruction (ACLR) after an ACL tear. Black and Hispanic youth have a more significant surgical delay to ACLR, increased risk for loss to clinical follow-up, and fewer physical therapy sessions, thereby leading to more significant deficits in knee extensor strength during rehabilitation. Furthermore, they found that Hispanic and Black patients had a higher risk of hospital admission after ACLR. Women have higher rates of ACL injury, with inconclusive evidence on the anatomic predisposition and ACL failure rate differences between genders.

In recent literature, several investigators have found inferior return to sports and functional outcomes following ACLR in women.[27,33] In addition, the investigators suggest disparities in those who undergo ACLR and their time to treatment. Other investigators have found that sex-based outcomes differ after ACL reconstruction depending on the used metric.[34]

DISCUSSION

Unconscious bias originates from patterns humans develop from the ability to create configurations in small bits of information. These configurations emerge from positive and negative attitudes and stereotypes people unconsciously develop about certain situations and individuals. This cognitive process generates a behavioral pattern that evolves from unconscious biases and helps to sort and filter people's perceptions. Moreover, it promotes inconsistent decision-making and possible systematic errors in judgment.[35]

Health care professionals have the same level of implicit bias as the general population, and higher levels are linked with suboptimal quality care. Providers with higher levels of bias are more likely to demonstrate unequal treatment recommendations, disparities in pain management, and even a lack of empathy toward minority patients.[36]

HOW DO WE TACKLE THE PRESENCE AND UNCONSCIOUS RESPONSE OF IMPLICIT BIAS DURING ATHLETE'S CARE?

I. Strategies for the application of strategies for future conversations and experiences with athletes
   - Existing implicit bias mitigation techniques

Education and self-awareness about the presence of implicit bias and its potentially harmful effects on judgment and behavior may lead individuals to pursue corrective action and mitigation.[37] Mitigation is defined as the action to reduce or exclude the occurrence of an undesirable event.[38] Implicit bias can be mitigated with awareness and effective bias-reduction strategies. Implicit bias mitigation aims to generate awareness of an individual's unconscious bias and related actions to consciously redirect our response and decision-making process. According to several investigators, effective communication strategies reduce implicit bias.[1] In addition, many of these strategies can be applied to mitigate implicit bias during athlete interventions.

- Devine and colleagues published 6 strategies to reduce unconscious bias[1]:
  1. Stereotype replacement
     i. Recognize that a response is based on a stereotype and is consciously adjusting the response.
  2. Counterstereotypic imaging
     i. The exercise of imagining the individual as the opposite of the stereotype.
  3. Individuation
     i. Seeing the person as an individual rather than a stereotype.
  4. Perspective taking
     i. Putting yourself in the other person's shoes.

5. Increasing opportunities
    i. Increase occasions for contact with individuals from different groups.
    ii. It is expanding one's network of friends and colleagues.
    iii. Contemplate attending events with people of other racial and ethnic groups, gender identities, sexual orientations, and other groups.
6. Partnership building
    i. Intend reframing the interaction with the patient as one between collaborating equals rather than between a high and low status.

- Augustus and colleagues published the book "*Seeing Patients: Unconscious Bias in Health Care*" and expressed practical tips to combat implicit bias in the health care field[39]:
  1. Understanding culture
     a. The team physician must have a basic understanding of the cultures of the athlete.
  2. Avoid stereotyping
     a. Avoid stereotyping the athlete and individuating them by consciously avoiding unconscious bias.
  3. Understand unconscious bias
     a. The team physician must comprehend the power of unconscious bias. Recognizing the personal triggers and consciously avoiding their influence in the decision-making process help mitigate the power of unconscious bias. There is an association between a more substantial implicit bias and poorer patient-provider communication.
     b. The Implicit Association Test enables measurements of implicit bias automatic associations between concepts. It measures the strength of association between notions, evaluations, and stereotypes. This test helps to identify the team physician's own unconscious bias. The test assesses if mental links exist between concepts and potentially associated values. The main idea is that making a response is more straightforward when closely related items share the same response key.[22]
  4. Recognize
     a. Recognize situations that magnify stereotyping and bias.
  5. Culturalization
     a. Know the national culturally and linguistically appropriate services standards.
  6. Teach Back
     a. Do a "Teach Back" method to confirm patient understanding of health care instructions associated with improved adherence, quality, and patient safety.
  7. Practice evidence-based medicine
     a. Assiduously practice evidence-based medicine.
- Several investigators have expressed their strategies to mitigate implicit bias.[40–44] The most important of these strategies include the following:
  - Perspective-taking[42]
    - Imagine being the person who experiences people questioning your ability or skills because of your social identity.
  - Counterstereotypic examples[40]
    - Identify scientists of diverse backgrounds in your field.
    - Implicit stereotypes are malleable, and controlled processes, such as mental imagery, influence the stereotyping process at its early and later stages.

- Interrupt automatic biased thoughts[45]
  - Identify when a person is influenced by implicit bias and helps create a response-conscious action plan. Therefore, implementation intentions may be an effective and efficient means of controlling automatic thought aspects.
- Education[41,46]
  - Carnes and colleagues[41]
    - An intervention that facilitates intentional behavioral change can help faculty break the gender bias habit and change department climate in ways that should support women's career advancement in academic medicine, science, and engineering.
  - Girod and colleagues[44]
    - Providing education on bias and strategies for reducing it can serve as an essential step toward reducing gender bias in academic medicine and, ultimately, promoting institutional change, specifically promoting women to higher ranks.

Communication strategies during athlete intervention and care

The first step in preventing implicit bias is educating ourselves about the spontaneous cognitive processes that unconsciously affect our clinical decisions. In 2019, Edgoose and colleagues recommended 3 primary strategies to mitigate implicit bias: educate, expose, and approach (**Fig. 1**). Furthermore, these strategies were subdivided into 8 evidence-based tactics.[35]

1. EDUCATE
   a. Introspection:
      i. Take the Implicit Association Test to recognize
         1. This test measures the strength of associations between concepts (eg, black people, gay people) and evaluations (eg, good, bad) or stereotypes (eg, athletic, clumsy). The main idea is that making a response is more straightforward when closely related items share the same response key.[46]
      ii. Confront and explore your own implicit biases.
   b. Mindfulness
      i. Increasing mindfulness improves our coping ability and modifies biological reactions that influence attention, emotional regulation, and habit formation.[47]
2. EXPOSE
   a. Expose to counterstereotypes and focus on the unique individuals you interact with.

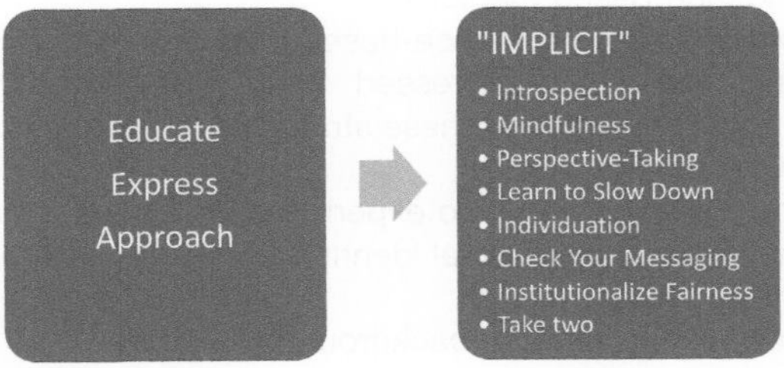

Fig. 1. Strategies to combat our implicit biases.[38] (*From*: Edgoose JYC, Quiogue M, and Sidhar K. How to Identify, Understand, and Unlearn Implicit Bias in Patient Care. Fam Pract Manag, 2019. 26(4): p. 29-33.)

   b. Avoid similarity and experience bias.
      Exposure to other groups and ways of thinking can help mitigate the similarity and experience bias.
   c. Perspective-talking
   d. Learn to slow down
      i. Acknowledging the potential for bias is crucial for the physician to recognize that safe options remain for managing patients' conditions.
   e. Individuation
      i. This method relies on gathering specific information about the person interrelating with you to counteract group-based stereotypic inferences.
3. APPROACH
   a. Check your messaging
      i. Using specific messages designed to create a more inclusive environment and mitigate implicit bias can make a real difference. For example, statements that welcome and embrace multiculturalism will have more success in decreasing unconscious bias.

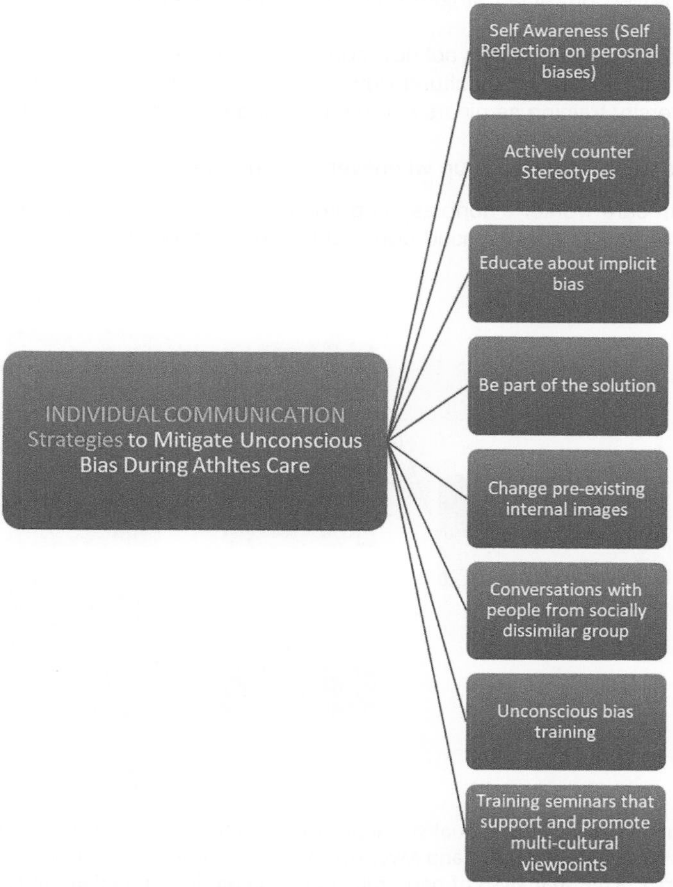

Fig. 2. Individual communication strategies for athlete's interventions and health care.

b. Institutionalize fairness
   i. Organizations are responsible for supporting a culture of diversity and inclusion because individual actions are not enough to deconstruct systemic inequities.
c. Take two
   i. Implicit bias mitigation strategies require constant revision and reflection during an individual's cultural transformation.

- Checklist for recognizing and minimizing the influence of implicit bias**Fig. 2**
  - Acknowledge biases in yourself and others.
  - Simply knowing about implicit bias and its potentially harmful effects on judgment and behavior may prompt individuals to pursue corrective action.
  - Be part of the solution.
  - Be self-aware.
  - Frequently evaluate your judgments for the influence of unconscious bias.
  - Change potential preexisting internal images.
  - Have conversations with people from socially distinct groups and focus on what you need to learn to grow.
  - Unconscious bias training produces better workplace environments, improved physician athlete-relationship and communication, and improved care outcomes.
  - Training seminars that acknowledge and promote an appreciation of group differences and multicultural viewpoints can help reduce implicit bias.[48]
  - Diversity training seminars can be a starting point for cultural change.[49]
  - Raise awareness
  - Recognize and speak up whenever you observe unconscious bias.

The health care worker's nonbiased approach to athlete care: transform bias from biased-unconscious to nonbiased-conscious.[48] As a leader and a team physician,

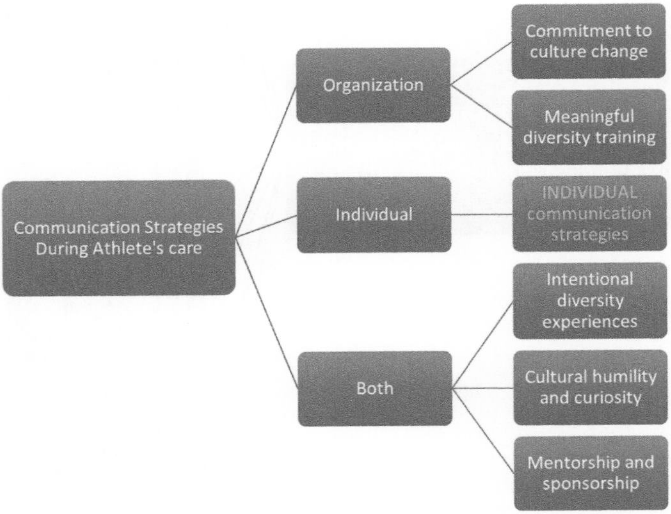

Fig. 3. Organization and individual strategies to mitigate unconscious bias during athlete care. (*From*: Hewett TE, Ford KR, and Myer GD. Anterior cruciate ligament injuries in female athletes: Part 2, a meta-analysis of neuromuscular interventions aimed at injury prevention. Am J Sports Med, 2006. 34(3): p. 490-8.)

use inclusive language, increase diversity to include underrepresented groups on the team, and make efforts to empower everyone equally and support underrepresented groups. Encourage leadership to offer training and workshops on unconscious bias.

SUMMARY

Unconscious bias, also known as implicit bias, is the principal contributor to the perpetuation of discrimination[1–4] and is a robust determinant of behavior because people lack personal awareness of them. They can happen despite conscious nonprejudiced intentions[1,5,7,10] due to an automatic and unconscious response. These unconscious and hidden biases may interfere with the actions and behaviors of the reflective and conscious side.[6]

Education and self-awareness about implicit bias and its potentially harmful effects on judgment and behavior drive individuals to pursue corrective action and mitigation.[37] Moreover, it is paramount that individuals seek corrective actions and mitigation strategies to improve team physician-athlete relationships, athlete performance, and care.

It is vital to mitigate and transform ethnic disparities into a provider's desire to avoid unconscious bias, resulting in the best possible care for patients.[3,40] During athlete interventions, team physicians must consider not only race and gender but also critical social determinants of health, access to care, and patient expectations, all of which can significantly affect patient outcomes.[27] In addition, individuals must become conscious and aware of their biases to act and redirect their responses.

Organizations and individuals must consistently create protocols to follow existing implicit bias mitigation and communication strategies. Furthermore, follow guidelines that implement the necessary changes to begin an evolution and consciously identify and change the automatic preferences that drive their judgment and decision-making. As shown in **Fig. 3**, there are already published strategies and infrastructure for organizations and individuals to help mitigate unconscious bias during patient interventions and athlete care. Furthermore, **Fig. 2** provides specific individuals' strategies to reduce unconscious bias and improve patients' and athletes' health care outcomes.

The interaction, communication, and care of athletes are also affected by implicit bias. Therefore, it is paramount to follow implicit bias mitigation and communication strategies to improve the outcome of athletes' intervention and care (see **Fig. 1**).

With sufficient motivation, cognitive resources, and effort, the team physician can focus on the unique qualities of the athletes, rather than on the groups they belong to, in forming impressions and behaving toward others. Furthermore, it is paramount to mitigate and transform ethnic disparities into a provider's desire to avoid unconscious bias, resulting in the best care for athletes.

CLINICS CARE POINTS

- Implicit race biases are the principal contributor to the perpetuation of discrimination.[1–4]
- Unconscious bias occurs spontaneously and unintentionally, affecting the judgment, decision-making, outcomes, and athlete's care.[1,5]
- The mind has an automatic or unconscious side and the reflective or conscious side. Hidden biases are a by-product of the unconscious side and may interfere with the actions and behaviors of the reflective and conscious side.[37]
- Implicit biases persist and are robust determinants of behavior because people lack personal awareness of them, and they can happen despite conscious nonprejudiced intentions.[1,4,12]

- "Humans possess mental blindspots like our visual blind spots—they exist without conscious awareness." "These blindspots house our hidden biases, or 'mind bugs,' which directly conflict with our conscious beliefs and ideologies".[4]
- Implicit attitudes are often significantly related to patient-provider interactions and health outcomes than treatment processes.[5]
- Education and self-awareness about implicit bias are paramount to swift individuals to pursue corrective actions and mitigation strategies to improve team physician-athlete relationships, athlete's performance, well-being, and care.[6]
- It is paramount to mitigate and transform ethnic disparities into a provider's desire to avoid unconscious bias, resulting in the best possible care for patients.[3,40]
- It is also known as unconscious bias, is often automatically activated, and operates at a level below consciousness. It is an unconscious preference in judgment and behavior that results from subtle cognitive processes.[9]
- When health care providers understand that stereotyping and racial prejudice are regular aspects of human cognition, they are more open to learning about this phenomenon and how it affects medical practice.[30]
- Health care professionals have the same level of implicit bias as the general population, and higher levels are linked with suboptimal quality care.[36]
- Providers with higher levels of bias are more likely to demonstrate unequal treatment recommendations, disparities in pain management, and even a lack of empathy toward minority patients.[8,9,36]
- Effective communication strategies reduce implicit bias.[1]
- Education and self-awareness about implicit bias and its potentially harmful effects on judgment and behavior may lead individuals to pursue corrective action and mitigation.[6,37,40]
- Three primary strategies to mitigate implicit bias: Educate, Expose, and Approach.[35]
- Training seminars that acknowledge and promote an appreciation of group differences and multicultural viewpoints can help reduce implicit bias.[48]
- Diversity training seminars can be a starting point for cultural change.[49]
- The health care worker's nonbiased approach to athlete care: transform bias from biased-unconscious to nonbiased-conscious.[8,48]
- During athlete interventions, team physicians must consider not only race and gender but also critical social determinants of health, access to care, and patient expectations, all of which can significantly affect patient outcomes.[27]
- Both organizations and individuals must create protocols and guidelines that implement changes to begin an evolution to consciously identify and change the automatic preferences that drive their judgment and decision-making.
- Developing implicit bias mitigation and communication strategies to improve the health care professional's outcome with athletes is paramount.

DISCLOSURE

P.J. Tort; Consultant for Exactech, Smith, and Nephew, and Conmed.

REFERENCES

1. Devine PG, et al. Long-term reduction in implicit race bias: A prejudice habit-breaking intervention. J Exp Soc Psychol 2012;48(6):1267–78.

2. Dovidio JF, Gaertner SL. Aversive racism and selection decisions: 1989 and 1999. Psychol Sci 2000;11(4):315–9.
3. Friske ST, Lln M. The contlnuum model: ten years later. In: Trope SCY, editor. Dual process Theories in social psychology. 1999. p. 211–54.
4. Gaertner SL, Dovidio JF. The aversive form of racism. In: Dovidio JF, Gaertner SL, editors. Prejudice, discrimination, and racism. Orlando, FL: Academic Press; 1986. p. 61–89.
5. Hall WJ, et al. Implicit Racial/Ethnic Bias Among Health Care Professionals and Its Influence on Health Care Outcomes: A Systematic Review. Am J Public Health 2015;105(12):e60–76.
6. Mahzarin Banaji, A.G., Blindspot: Hidden Biases of Good People. 2013.
7. Greenwald AG, Banaji MR. Implicit social cognition: attitudes, self-esteem, and stereotypes. Psychol Rev 1995;102(1):4–27.
8. Dasgupta N, Greenwald AG. On the malleability of automatic attitudes: combating automatic prejudice with images of admired and disliked individuals. J Pers Soc Psychol 2001;81(5):800–14.
9. Team, I.M., How to Reduce Implicit Bias. 2017: p. 1-4.
10. Allen R, McConnell J. Relations among the Implicit Association Test, Discriminatory Behavior, and Explicit Measures of Racial Attitudes. J Exp Soc Psychol 2001;435–42.
11. Bertrand M. Are Emily and Greg more employable than Lakisha and Jamal? Am Econ Rev 2004;94.
12. Bargh, J.A., The cognitive monster: The case against the controllability of automatic stereotype effects. 1999: p. 361-382.
13. Lighthall GK, Vazquez-Guillamet C. Understanding Decision Making in Critical Care. Clin Med Res 2015;13(3–4):156–68.
14. Rebecca Blank, C., Hiring the best and brightest: Understanding unconscious bias and improving our hiring practices and decisions. 2016.
15. Haider AH, et al. Racial disparities in surgical care and outcomes in the United States: a comprehensive review of patient, provider, and systemic factors. J Am Coll Surg 2013;216(3):482–92.e12.
16. Howell EA. Reducing Disparities in Severe Maternal Morbidity and Mortality. Clin Obstet Gynecol 2018;61(2):387–99.
17. Bass AR, et al. Higher Total Knee Arthroplasty Revision Rates Among United States Blacks Than Whites: A Systematic Literature Review and Meta-Analysis. J Bone Joint Surg Am 2016;98(24):2103–8.
18. Hawkins K, et al. Disparities in major joint replacement surgery among adults with Medicare supplement insurance. Popul Health Manag 2011;14(5):231–8.
19. Sanford Z, et al. Racial Disparities in Surgical Outcomes After Spine Surgery: An ACS-NSQIP Analysis. Global Spine J 2019;9(6):583–90.
20. Singh JA, Ramachandran R. Racial disparities in total ankle arthroplasty utilization and outcomes. Arthritis Res Ther 2015;17(1):70.
21. Skinner J, et al. Racial, ethnic, and geographic disparities in rates of knee arthroplasty among Medicare patients. N Engl J Med 2003;349(14):1350–9.
22. Maina IW, et al. A decade of studying implicit racial/ethnic bias in healthcare providers using the implicit association test. Soc Sci Med 2018;199:219–29.
23. Agel J, Rockwood T, Klossner D. Collegiate ACL Injury Rates Across 15 Sports: National Collegiate Athletic Association Injury Surveillance System Data Update (2004-2005 Through 2012-2013). Clin J Sport Med 2016;26(6):518–23.

24. Arendt E, Dick R. Knee injury patterns among men and women in collegiate basketball and soccer. NCAA data and review of literature. Am J Sports Med 1995;23(6):694–701.
25. Hewett TE, Ford KR, Myer GD. Anterior cruciate ligament injuries in female athletes: Part 2, a meta-analysis of neuromuscular interventions aimed at injury prevention. Am J Sports Med 2006;34(3):490–8.
26. Stracciolini A, et al. Female Sport Participation Effect on Long-Term Health-Related Quality of Life. Clin J Sport Med 2020;30(6):526–32.
27. Devana SK, et al. Disparities in ACL Reconstruction: the Influence of Gender and Race on Incidence, Treatment, and Outcomes. Curr Rev Musculoskelet Med 2022;15(1):1–9.
28. Poma PA. Race/Ethnicity Concordance Between Patients and Physicians. J Natl Med Assoc 2017;109(1):6–8.
29. Saha S, et al. Patient-physician racial concordance and the perceived quality and use of health care. Arch Intern Med 1999;159(9):997–1004.
30. Walker KO, Moreno G, Grumbach K. The association among specialty, race, ethnicity, and practice location among California physicians in diverse specialties. J Natl Med Assoc 2012;104(1–2):46–52.
31. Burgess D, et al. Reducing racial bias among health care providers: lessons from social-cognitive psychology. J Gen Intern Med 2007;22(6):882–7.
32. Druckman JN, et al. Racial bias in sport medical staff's perceptions of others' pain. J Soc Psychol 2018;158(6):721–9.
33. Tan SH, et al. The Importance of Patient Sex in the Outcomes of Anterior Cruciate Ligament Reconstructions: A Systematic Review and Meta-analysis. Am J Sports Med 2016;44(1):242–54.
34. Mok AC, et al. Sex-Specific Outcomes After Anterior Cruciate Ligament Reconstruction: A Systematic Review and Meta-analysis. Orthop J Sports Med 2022; 10(2). 23259671221076883.
35. Edgoose JYC, Quiogue M, Sidhar K. How to Identify, Understand, and Unlearn Implicit Bias in Patient Care. Fam Pract Manag 2019;26(4):29–33.
36. FitzGerald C, Hurst S. Implicit bias in healthcare professionals: a systematic review. BMC Med Ethics 2017;18(1):19.
37. Time TE. What is 'Mitigation. The Economics Time; 2022.
38. White AA, White AA, Chanoff D. Seeing patients: unconscious bias in health care. MA, USA/ London, England: Harvard University Press; 2011.
39. Blair IV, Steiner JF, Havranek EP. Unconscious (implicit) bias and health disparities: where do we go from here? Perm J 2011;15(2):71–8.
40. Green AR, et al. Implicit bias among physicians and its prediction of thrombolysis decisions for black and white patients. J Gen Intern Med 2007;22(9):1231–8.
41. Carnes M, et al. The effect of an intervention to break the gender bias habit for faculty at one institution: a cluster randomized, controlled trial. Acad Med 2015;90(2):221–30.
42. Galinsky AD, Moskowitz GB. Perspective-taking: decreasing stereotype expression, stereotype accessibility, and in-group favoritism. J Pers Soc Psychol 2000; 78(4):708–24.
43. Galinsky AD, Ku G. The effects of perspective-taking on prejudice: the moderating role of self-evaluation. Pers Soc Psychol Bull 2004;30(5):594–604.
44. Girod S, et al. Reducing Implicit Gender Leadership Bias in Academic Medicine With an Educational Intervention. Acad Med 2016;91(8):1143–50.

45. Stewart BD, Payne BK. Bringing automatic stereotyping under control: implementation intentions as efficient means of thought control. Pers Soc Psychol Bull 2008;34(10):1332–45.
46. De Houwer J. The Implicit Association Test as a tool for studying dysfunctional associations in psychopathology: strengths and limitations. J Behav Ther Exp Psychiatry 2002;33(2):115–33.
47. Burgess DJ, Beach MC, Saha S. Mindfulness practice: A promising approach to reducing the effects of clinician implicit bias on patients. Patient Educ Couns 2017;100(2):372–6.
48. Hammond MEH, et al. Bias in Medicine: Lessons Learned and Mitigation Strategies. JACC Basic Transl Sci 2021;6(1):78–85.
49. Brewer MB. A dual process model of impression formation. In: Srull T, Wyer RS, editors. Advances in social cognition 1988;1–36.

Section III: Putting it together for a better future

The Intrinsic Value of Diversity in Team Leadership

Chase Gauthier, MD, Justin Kung, MD, Jeffrey Guy, MD*

KEYWORDS

• Diversity • Leadership • Communication • Problem-solving • Inspiration

KEY POINTS

- Diversity within leadership groups allows for more effective communication with team members, thereby creating stronger bonds and allowing team members to reach their full potential.
- Successful relationships are built on trust. Diversity within leadership is necessary for increasing the trust between team members and leadership.
- Diversity allows leadership groups to expand their potential solutions to a given issue, which grants a greater likelihood of choosing the optimal solution.
- Displaying diversity in leadership positions is important for inspiring those from similar backgrounds, thereby ensuring future diversity within leadership groups and optimal team functioning.

INTRODUCTION

Each year, the United States becomes more diverse, with current estimates suggesting this trend will continue into the coming years.[1,2] As such, diversity within workforces has also grown, with studies demonstrating that this increase in diversity among workers has a positive effect on the efficiency and quality of the work produced.[3] In academic institutions, specifically, the concept of diversity and inclusion has grown in popularity in recent years. Diversity within a health care team structure has also been demonstrated to have a positive effect on the work produced by the team, with patients having improved patient outcomes and more ethical and equitable care when treated by a health care team composed of diverse persons.[3–7] Despite this demonstrated effect in team settings, how diversity effects those in leadership positions has not been fully researched simply due to the lack of diversity in leadership within professional organizations.[8–12] This article will highlight the importance of diversity among leadership positions, demonstrate ways in which diversity among leadership can directly lead to positive team outcomes, and make a claim for why diversity should be a core concept

Department of Orthopedic Surgery, Prisma Health, 2 Medical Park Road, Suite 404, Columbia, SC 29203, USA
* Corresponding author.
E-mail address: jadgdr@aol.com

Clin Sports Med 43 (2024) 293–297
https://doi.org/10.1016/j.csm.2023.12.001
sportsmed.theclinics.com
0278-5919/24/

of effective leadership teams, similar to the way attributes such as an adequate knowledge base and honesty are necessary to be an effective leader.

DIVERSITY IN COMMUNICATION

One of the most fundamental, yet overlooked, aspects of an effective leader is the ability to connect with team members in a truly meaningful way. This ability to communicate and connect with team members is necessary for developing a bond between a leader and the person they lead. Diversity among leadership positions helps to facilitate these bonds through the broadening of certain aspects of communication. This can include increasing the amount of inclusive language used when communicating with members of a team and creating more identity-concordant interactions, which may improve overall communication.[13] Diversity within leadership also brings diversity in communication styles, which may also benefit team interactions through the avoidance of "communication blind spots" or discordance in communication style between 2 parties. Although a certain leader might not be able to effectively communicate with a given member of a team, in a properly diverse leadership group, it is more likely that someone else may be able to understand the optimal way to connect with that member. By interacting with these other leaders and developing a greater ability to identify and correct communication blind spots, one can learn the optimal way to connect with a greater proportion of team members than would have been possible otherwise. With diversity as a central component of a leadership group, whether in sports or a career setting, proper communication among all team members may be achieved and the team may reach their full potential.

DIVERSITY IN TRUST

At the core of any relationship, whether it be between a coach and his players, a team physician and his team, or an owner and his workers, is trust. Trust is fundamental to building a successful professional and therapeutic relationship, with trust between coaching staff, players, and ownership being central to any successful sports organization. Similarities between a leader and team members influence the development of that trust, as recent studies have demonstrated persons of color were more likely to be receptive to recommendations by a physician if that physician was also a person of color.[13,14] However, leadership in sports organizations, including coaching staff and team physicians, are generally not as diverse as the players in which they lead and provide care.[12,15,16] Players who have particular life experiences, therefore, might gravitate toward and ultimately trust coaches who have similar life experiences. In a situation where there is limited diversity among a coaching staff, it may take longer, and leadership staff may have to extend more effort to build a trusting relationship with players with diverse lived experiences, which may ultimately affect the success of the team. Therefore, diversity within leadership positions, including coaching staff, team physicians, general managers, and owners, is necessary to help build trust between players and their organization's leadership, which is important for the organization to be successful. Within medicine, as well, diversity among health care teams is necessary to build trust within a patient-physician relationship, which in turn can have a positive impact on patient health and overall satisfaction with their care.

DIVERSITY IN PROBLEM-SOLVING

An additional important skill that any leader ought to possess is the ability to address potential issues that may arise in a group setting. The ability to problem-solve as issues arise as well as foresee potential conflict is the direct result of learned experiences throughout one's life, as one will view a problem and its potential solutions from a perspective based upon their own experience. If 10 members of a given leadership team are of similar backgrounds with similar learned experiences, they will think of a problem in the same light and, as such, will develop a narrower set of solutions. If 10 members of a leadership team are from different backgrounds, however, they are more likely to think of the problem from different angles and, in turn, can develop a much wider variety of solutions based on their individual perspectives. This expansion of potential answers to problems can be crucial in facilitating the overall success of a team, as each problem may require a wide variety of options to be discussed to determine the overall best solution.

If a leadership group does not have the diversity necessary to develop multiple varied solutions to a given problem, it will inevitably run into a situation in which the optimal solution is not considered and, as such, the team will not achieve its best. To further illustrate this concept, consider interprofessional rounding, which has occurred with greater frequency in recent years within many hospital systems. This type of rounding works by bringing together those from multiple educational backgrounds to treat patient care more holistically. Similarly, differences in life experiences within a leadership team will provide a more holistic approach to issues that arise. As such, the chances of determining the optimal solution will be greatly increased compared to if there were no differing life experiences within the leadership group.

DIVERSITY IN INSPIRATION

Although in some ways cliché, the visibility of persons with diverse backgrounds in leadership roles is important in igniting inspiration and drive and eventually in facilitating the development of those from similar backgrounds. Seeing another person from a similar cultural, racial, or gender background move past the "glass ceiling," an unofficial barrier in professional advancement that tends to affect women and persons of color, into a prominent leadership position may, in turn, inspire others of a similar background. Goals are ultimately achieved through a combination of dedication and inspiration, and those in leadership positions often find themselves in an optimal position to inspire others. As such, it is important that people of differing backgrounds see people they can relate to in prominent leadership positions to encourage them and demonstrate that they too are capable and welcome in similar types of leadership roles.

As stated previously, diversity in leadership roles is necessary for optimal functioning in a team setting. As such, it is important to provide opportunities and a roadmap to those of varying backgrounds detailing the process of obtaining and succeeding in these leadership positions. Without this, younger generations may be less likely, through lack of encouragement or perceived unattainability, to progress forward and may not reach a stage to even be considered for leadership roles, which will inevitably hinder the overall ability of a team and possibly prevent the team from being able to provide the best possible outcomes. Therefore, highlighting leaders from diverse backgrounds is important to inspire and provide guidance for future generations, so they may feel fully capable of developing the skills necessary to be effective leaders who can promote the best possible team functioning.

It is clear from the previously stated information that diversity within leadership teams allows for more productive and inclusive functioning, which ultimately can produce superior results compared to leadership teams that lack diversity. An organization's ultimate goal is to be successful. Therefore, organizations, whether they be health care systems or sports teams, should emphasize the creation of diverse leadership teams to grow in a positive direction and be successful.

SUMMARY

The central question posed by this article concerns why diversity is important in leadership positions in a variety of settings, from professional groups to sports to health care. This article has highlighted the many ways diversity is necessary for optimal team function, including diversity among communication styles, the ability to connect with team members in a way that is most meaningful to them, diversity in perspectives for addressing problems, and the subsequent variety in potential solutions, and how the optics of diverse leadership inspire future generations to achieve similar leadership positions, thereby ensuring diversity in leadership and optimal team function for years to come. Overall, diverse leadership teams simply will perform better and be more successful than leadership teams that are not diverse. It is, therefore, clear that there is observable value in constructing a diverse leadership group for any team and, as such, organizations should strive to promote diversity in the interest of broadening their abilities and overall potential.

CLINICS CARE POINTS

- Diversity within team leadership may help increase a team's overall potential and is an important consideration in creating leadership teams.
- Diversity within team leadership may improve the communication, trust, and problem-solving skills of a team.

DISCLOSURE

The authors have no conflicts of interest to disclose.

REFERENCES

1. Jensen E, Jones N, Rabe M, et al. 2020 U.S. Population More Racially and Ethnically Diverse Than Measured in 2010. Available at: https://www.census.gov/library/stories/2021/08/2020-united-states-population-more-racially-ethnically-diverse-than-2010.html. Accessed November 27, 2023.
2. Vespa J., Medina L., Armstron D.M., Demographic Turning Points for the United States: Population Projections for 2020 to 2060. Available at: https://www.census.gov/content/dam/Census/library/publications/2020/demo/p25-1144.pdf. Accessed November 27, 2023.
3. Gomez LE, Bernet P. Diversity improves performance and outcomes. Journal of the National Medical Association 2019;111(4):383–92.
4. LaVeist TA, Pierre G. Integrating the 3Ds–social determinants, health disparities, and health-care workforce diversity. Public Health Rep 2014;129(Suppl 2):9–14.
5. Bradley EH. Diversity, Inclusive Leadership, and Health Outcomes. Int J Health Policy Manag 2020;1. https://doi.org/10.15171/ijhpm.2020.12.
6. Cobianchi L, Dal Mas F, Massaro M, et al. Diversity and ethics in trauma and acute care surgery teams: results from an international survey. World J Emerg Surg 2022;17(1):44.

7. Curry LA, Brault MA, Linnander EL, et al. Influencing organisational culture to improve hospital performance in care of patients with acute myocardial infarction: a mixed-methods intervention study. BMJ Qual Saf 2018;27(3):207–17.
8. Lerman C, Hughes-Halbert C, Falcone M, et al. Leadership Diversity and Development in the Nation's Cancer Centers. JNCI: Journal of the National Cancer Institute 2022;114(9):1214–21.
9. Sanghavi R, Reisch J, Tomer G. Diversity in Selected Leadership Positions in United States Academic Pediatric Gastroenterology Programs: A Review and Call to Action. J Pediatr Gastroenterol Nutr 2022;74(2):244–7.
10. Sossou CW, Fakhra S, Batra K, et al. Diversity in U.S. Cardiovascular Trainees and Leadership Where we are and What the Future Holds. Curr Probl Cardiol 2023;48(3):101518.
11. Mattson LM, Rosario-Concepcion RA, Hurdle MFB, et al. Gender Diversity in Primary Care Sports Medicine Leadership. Curr Sports Med Rep 2022;21(8):303–8.
12. Lapchick R.E., 2022 Racial and Gender Report Card. In: Ervin A., Franks L., Gregory D., et al, editors. Available at: https://www.tidesport.org/_files/ugd/ac4087_31b60a6a51574cbe9b552831c0fcbd3f.pdf. Accessed November 27, 2023.
13. Shen MJ, Peterson EB, Costas-Muñiz R, et al. The Effects of Race and Racial Concordance on Patient-Physician Communication: A Systematic Review of the Literature. J Racial and Ethnic Health Disparities 2018;5(1):117–40.
14. Saha S, Beach MC. Impact of Physician Race on Patient Decision-Making and Ratings of Physicians: a Randomized Experiment Using Video Vignettes. J Gen Intern Med 2020;35(4):1084–91.
15. Wiggins AJ, Agha O, Diaz A, et al. Current Perceptions of Diversity Among Head Team Physicians and Head Athletic Trainers: Results Across US Professional Sports Leagues. Orthopaedic Journal of Sports Medicine 2021;9(10). 232596712110472.
16. Wilson J, Agha O, Wiggins AJ, et al. Gender and Racial Diversity Among the Head Medical and Athletic Training Staff of Women's Professional Sports Leagues. Orthopaedic Journal of Sports Medicine 2023;11(2). 232596712211504.

Diversity, Equity, and Inclusion Leadership

A True Team Sport

Erica Taylor, MD, MBA

KEYWORDS

• Leadership • Strategy • Teams • Inclusion • Diversity • Playbook • Metrics

KEY POINTS

- To elevate and sustain diversity, equity, and inclusion (DEI) leadership, organizations should lean into a deeper understanding of the nuances of leading the efforts of this complex movement.
- Team members need to be aligned on mission and vision as a critical first step to harnessing the power of diversity and inclusion.
- Leaders shouldcreate value around the team that is visible and understood by supporters within and external to the environment.
- Intentional metrics that qualify and quantify various aspects of equity and inclusion must be created to capture the meaningful impact of DEI efforts.
- The actions of creating a strategic plan and working together to form your unique playbook can foster cohesion and honest introspection that is more valuable than the actual end-product of a plan.

THE COMPLEXITY OF A LEADERSHIP MOVEMENT

There is more dynamic engagement within the areas of diversity, equity, and inclusion (DEI) in orthopedic surgery today than ever before. In addition, over the recent years, health care and corporate institutions alike have approached culture evolution from multiple pathways. For example, many academic departments and companies worked to designate an individual to serve as a DEI leader. In response to the increased emphasis on combating societal injustices and health-related disparities that has occurred since 2020, the rate of appointment of DEI leaders increased dramatically. However, the suboptimal structure and support of this specific leadership position and fatiguing engagement from any corresponding teams have limited

Duke Department of Orthopaedics Vice Chair of Equity, Diversity, and Inclusion & Orthopaedic Surgeon, Duke Health Integrated Practice CMO of Diversity, Equity, and Inclusion, Duke University School of Medicine, Duke Fuqua School of Business Executive in Residence Faculty, Orthopaedic Diversity Leadership Consortium, PO Box 1726, Wake Forest, NC 27587, USA
E-mail address: erica.taylor@orthodiversity.org

Clin Sports Med 43 (2024) 299–309
https://doi.org/10.1016/j.csm.2023.11.001
0278-5919/24/

the potential of this movement and, in several cases, have led to the turnover of the DEI leader and the dismantling of their teams.[1]

According to a review by the Orthopedic Diversity Leadership Consortium *(www.orthodiversity.org)*, there are at least three competing forces at play.[2] First, effective integration of DEI leadership and teams into traditional organization structure is not fully understood, with little precedent on how diversity-focused positions and committees are defined or supported. Second, while statistics on the low diversity in surgical fields are often published, there is a notable shortage of *solution-based* resources describing strategies to guide effective initiatives. Third, surgical care environments are multidisciplinary teams, bringing nurses, advanced practice providers, surgeons, technicians, learners, and anesthesiologists into a single setting with a complex, often high-stress culture. Promoting interprofessional collaboration that accounts for the diversity of the team is a critical yet undervalued leadership skill.

To mitigate these underlying challenges to effective, sustainable DEI leadership, organizations can lean into a deeper understanding of the nuances of this domain and explore the best ways to harness the power of having diverse teams on a system level.[3] This review will focus on the power of team dynamics when working toward goals of creating healthy, inclusive environments. The author will use parallels from sports to outline pragmatic steps to move forward.

THE POWER OF INTERPROFESSIONAL COLLABORATION

Taking care of patients has never been a solo sport. Leading DEI is not either. Our orthopedic surgical care environments are inherently multidisciplinary, incorporating team members from a variety of specialties and occupations. As such, the culture within surgery is complex and there are potential sources of implicit bias, resource disparity, interpersonal discourse, and isolation. If left unchecked, these culture threats can work against even the best of DEI efforts. A path forward is created when the power of having a variety of backgrounds, perspectives, and experiences aligned toward a common mission is cultivated within a healthy team. This is not an intuitive or easy task.

For many years, the benefits of interprofessional collaboration in health care have been highlighted. In 2010, the World Health Organization declared the essential need for collaborative clinical practice.[4] Recently, a research group published on validated frameworks for interprofessional collaboration, focusing on the core competencies that support and enhance the benefits of diverse teams working together.[5] A particularly popular framework cited in this study focused on "learning about, from, and with each other" while drawing on the strengths and capacities of team members.

As described earlier, there is power in numbers but only when those numbers are aligned and clear on the mission and vision. This can certainly be applied to DEI leadership and associated team empowerment. The following sections include guidelines that any DEI team, particularly those that are interprofessional, can use to improve effectiveness and sustainability of this critical work. Just as we have learned invaluable leadership lessons from the sports arena, we can also find numerous parallels to DEI leadership.

MOVING FORWARD: THE PLAYBOOK GUIDELINES

At this point, your organization may have already formed a DEI committee, task force, work group, or team. At minimum, the key stakeholders for change and target audiences have been identified. As in sports, it is possible that the leader and team members have been training for this work all their lives. Conversely, perhaps some of them were drafted. Or maybe some of them participated in aspects of DEI work in unofficial capacities earlier in their career paths and decided to take their contributions to the next level. Regardless of the origin story, the team is here, and the hope is that it is an inclusive interprofessional group that brings in perspectives from all different areas of your patient population served, as well as your internal culture. To achieve this optimal reality, there are 4 key elements in the DEI leadership playbook that should be followed.

I: Establish a Common Purpose

> *I get a group of people who are talented to commit to excellence and to work together as one. That's where it starts. Different talents, same commitment.*
>
> *—Michael Krzyzewski (American basketball coach)*

In any sports team, it is beneficial to understand the motivations and goals for each player. Indeed, the overall team may have stated mission and goals, but unless you recognize and achieve understanding of what motivated individuals to join a sport or a team in the first place, you may be setting yourselves up for failure. Some people join teams to win championships. Others join for an opportunity to do what they love and inspire others. Others participate because of the innumerable benefits to mental health. It may be all the aforementioned reasons. The combinations of possible motivations are numerous.

Similarly, when it comes to areas of diversity, equity, inclusion, and belonging, the list of potential areas of passion and focus is extensive. Often "DEI work" is used in an overly simplistic manner as if all DEI efforts are created equal and can be lumped together. In reality, the scope of DEI can be myopic, broad-reaching, or somewhere in between. **Box 1** lists examples of the variety of priority areas focused on by orthopedic DEI leaders, highlighting not only a diverse array of subject matter but also a diverse array of target populations. Is the team's goal recruitment and retention? Or is the team focused on health equity, defined as the state in which everyone has a fair and just opportunity to attain their highest level of health?[6] If recruitment and retention are key focus areas, which population is the target—students, graduate medical education trainees, faculty, staff, or executive leaders? Or something else altogether? Consider the complexity of establishing a common vision within recruitment alone.

As an early step, a functional DEI team will need to decide which areas will be the foundation of their mission, vision, and goal that all team members can agree upon. While all the potential domains are critical, understanding what universally motivates and creates energy for all team members will improve effectiveness. Further, understanding and validating the personal goals of each team member will create an important level of connectedness.

II: Create Value for the Team

> *Sport has the power to change the world. It has the power to inspire, the power to unite people in a way that little else does. It speaks to youth in a language they understand. Sports can create hope, where there was once only despair...It laughs in the face of all types of discrimination.*
>
> *—Nelson Mandela (Former President of South Africa and activist)*

Box 1
Sample list of potential areas of focus for diversity, equity, and inclusion leaders and teams:

Diversifying student-faculty pathways (ie, pipeline programs)

Diversity and inclusion in research and clinical trials

Gender equity and policies

Department/company climate and culture

LGBQTIA+ equity and policies

Inclusive search and hiring

Cultural competency education

Disability access and support

Supplier diversity

Community engagement

Racial/ethnic equity and policies

Health equity

Employee well-being

Employee resource groups (ie, affinity groups)

Abbreviation: LGBQTIA+, lesbian, gay, bisexual, queer or questioning, transgender, intersex, and asexual, or another diverse gender identity.

Now that you have created a team corralled together around common mission and goals, it is important to create value around the team that is visible and understood by supporters within and external to the environment. Across the board, sports teams bring value to spectators, fans, coaches, staff, and leagues in some way, shape, or form. Notably, the value is also felt by the teammates themselves. Even the smallest of teams can inspire and create a spark that warrants the time and ticket prices required to support.

Along the same lines, it is important to create value around and within a DEI leadership team. Historically, DEI effort was housed in a silo away from the organization's main goals and strategic priorities. It was considered volunteer work to be done outside of work hours and without resource support. Thus, the results from well-intentioned efforts were suboptimal, just as they would be for an unrecognized football team playing on unkempt turf and wearing below-regulation uniform padding without a coach.

Today, there is a pervasive call to action for organization leaders to swing the pendulum toward providing adequate resources to DEI leaders and diversity committees. Such resources can come in the form of dedicated time during the work week for team meetings, funding for initiatives and the leadership role, and promotional credit assigned for the members who are contributing to the organizational DEI goals. When these resources are not provided, there is a signal sent to the team and to the rest of the organization that these efforts are neither valuable nor valued. Such a sentiment would be contrary to the numerous studies that prove that there are a multitude of measurable value-added benefits from increasing diversity and belonging within an organization.

For example, in Scott Page's book, *The Diversity Bonus*, he presents the mathematical and practical bonuses of having heterogeneous teams when solving complex problems, such as those found in health care.[7] A groundbreaking report by McKinsey and Company outlined improved financial outperformance from companies with increased racial, ethnic, and gender diversity on their teams.[8] The higher the representation, the higher the likelihood of outperformance. Importantly, patient outcomes have also been improved when inclusion and equity have been embraced by healthcare teams.[9]

Moving away from the narrative that DEI effort is strictly volunteer work and an under-resourced burden is a necessary step forward. Specifically, identifying a wide variety of support, including designation of executive sponsors, and ascribing value to the leader and team will aid in effectiveness, relevance, and sustainability. The value proposition is clear and should be amplified to attract others to engage and contribute.

III: Measure Your Outputs... Inclusively

> *If winning isn't everything, why do they keep score?*
>
> *—Vince Lombardi (National Football League executive and coach)*

There is an age-old debate about whether keeping score in youth sports is a necessary part of teamwork and skill development or an unnecessary evil that can destroy self-confidence with very little to no benefit. Proponents of scorekeeping argue that keeping score promotes the development of the lifelong ability to cope with a miss or a loss. However, at the core, the purpose of having a score is not simply to determine who is winning and who is losing but rather to define measurements and goals that can be universally accepted as expectations.

In the DEI arena, having advanced metrics to define goals and expectations is surprisingly new. Traditional DEI goals barely measured any outcomes and, if they did, the focus was primarily on representation data. How many women are in a residency program? How many underrepresented minority physicians are in a practice? What percentage of researchers in a department identify a disability? For years, representation data have informed recruitment strategies, which in turn informed advancement initiatives, which then informed attrition mitigation methodology. And the cycle repeats. However, despite decades of emphasis on representation metrics, there continues to be significant disparity within orthopedics, and medicine in general, specifically in the areas of in pay equity, promotion, leadership enactment, inclusion and belonging, and resource allocation. In fact, there are fewer black men in medicine today than there were 40 years ago.[10]

So, why is not focusing solely on representation metrics enough? Well, just like the final score of a playoff game shows the outcome but not the heart and sweat displayed on the field, representation data alone do not give a holistic picture of the components of an environment that formulate a culture of belonging, equity, and respect. To truly investigate, understand, and then communicate a current state and measure trends, additional metrics must be incorporated in a thoughtful fashion. Start by looking at the data that are already collected in your organization and inquire whether demographic filters can be applied. For example, in our organization, the patient experience scores collected are housed in an easily accessed dashboard for each provider to review their individual reports. In 2021, a toggle field was created to apply various domains of demographic filters to assess for any relevant differences in communication and experience domains across populations. Modern culture surveys have incorporated intentional questions around belonging to assess whether employees and practitioners truly feel as if they can be authentic in the workplace.

Industries outside of health care have endorsed measuring community partnerships and total dollars invested in DEI initiatives.

Box 2 lists some examples of DEI metrics that may be relevant to your team, based on your common mission and goals and the value of DEI effort expected by your organization. Regardless of the metrics selected, ensure that (1) they are indeed measurable, (2) they cannot be artificially manipulated, and (3) they incentivize/promote desirable behaviors. The sweet spot combination of metrics should be relevant for your particular environment and will bring greater clarity and insight to your team's activities.

IV: Co-create Your Strategy

> *A lot of people notice when you succeed, but they don't see what it takes to get there.*
> *—Dawn Staley (American basketball player and coach)*

The official flag football arm of the National Football League created basic instructions for teams on how to create an effective playbook.[11] The instructional document identified the purpose of creating a playbook as a method of keeping a team's strategy consistent and organized from the beginning to help players build the fundamental skills necessary to have a successful season. In addition, they asserted that as players grew and gained confidence, the playbooks should be adapted, reorganized, and rearranged.

Box 2
Sample list of potential diversity, equity, and inclusion metrics topic areas:

Demographic representation in clinical teams

Demographic representation in senior leadership

Patient Experience Scores

Culture and Belonging Scores

Pay equity gap closure

Retention of clinicians and staff

Implementation of inclusive hiring practices

Community based organization partnerships

Minority-serving institutions/HBCU partnerships

Participation in professional development programs for underrepresented groups

Financial support for DEI leader and team resources

Resolution of professionalism complaints

Social determinants of health measures

Employee Well-Being Scores

Engagement of employee resource groups (ie, affinity groups)

Abbreviations: DEI, diversity, equity, and inclusion; HBCU, Historically Black Colleges and Universities.

This advisement rings true for determination of DEI strategy. It is tempting to ask a consulting group to provide a “copy and paste” strategic plan that will bring peace and harmony to all aspects of your organization. As discerned from the sections discussed earlier, this approach generally does not work. Each environment—and each team—will have a unique set of opportunities, a nuanced history, and a variety of characteristics that warrant a customized “playbook” be developed to achieve in the areas of DEI.

Indeed, foundational templates of a strategic plan are a great starting point for most organizations. However, the blanks should be filled in by the leadership and team members based on internal assessments and input from stakeholder groups. In fact, the act of creating a strategic plan and working together to form your unique playbook can foster cohesion and honest introspection that is more valuable than the actual end-product of a plan. As a first step, your team should understand what a strategic plan is and the benefit it provides. In a provocative article, business researcher Graham Kenny called out the reality that most strategic plans are not strategic and are likely not even plans.[12] He describes a common misinterpretation of “objectives” and “actions” as “strategy.” Understanding these important points can bring more intention to designing the plan that will help your group reach its DEI goals in a sustainable format.

Strategy creation technique: the KJ method

Whenever possible, co-create your strategic plan with the members of the DEI team and invite members of marginalized or underrepresented groups to participate as well. In 2022, our team utilized a unique methodology to help us identify and focus on relevant strategic priorities toward the future. Referred to as the “KJ Method,” or “KJ Technique” this approach to creating cohesive solutions was developed by Japanese ethnographer Jiro Kawakita.[13] This technique can be used by teams to generate ideas and identify priorities. As such, it is considered one of the most popular brainstorming exercises. There are 2 critical components to this exercise: creation of an *affinity diagram* and subsequent formation of an *intergraph.*

The steps for creation of an *affinity diagram* are outlined in **Fig. 1** and can be applied to any subject matter for a team, especially DEI. This is a proven technique for taking seemingly disjointed ideas and reframing them in an organized fashion. For this first stage of the exercise, teams are asked to individually identify key features of their optimal state, such as a diverse, inclusive, and equitable environment. The members of the group do this in silence, writing a single phrase or sentence on individual sticky notes. Once completed, the various notes are pasted to a board and the members can visualize all of the generated descriptors from their colleagues. If there are descriptors that are similar, such as “fair pay” and “pay equity,” those respective notes are grouped together. Hence, an affinity diagram is generated by the team with various groupings that are subsequently assigned agreed upon category labels (**Fig. 2**).

Once the affinity diagram is completed, the team will recognize that they have identified categories that represent the key components to achieve their optimal state of DEI. The team is now ready to create an *intergraph*, a graphic representation of the relationship between various priority categories. This is a powerful part of the experience, as the team evaluates each pair of categories and determines which category of a pair is the “driver” and which category is the “receiver.” For example, when comparing “diverse leadership” and “pay equity,” the group collectively decides which of the two categories drives the other. Does diverse leadership lead to pay

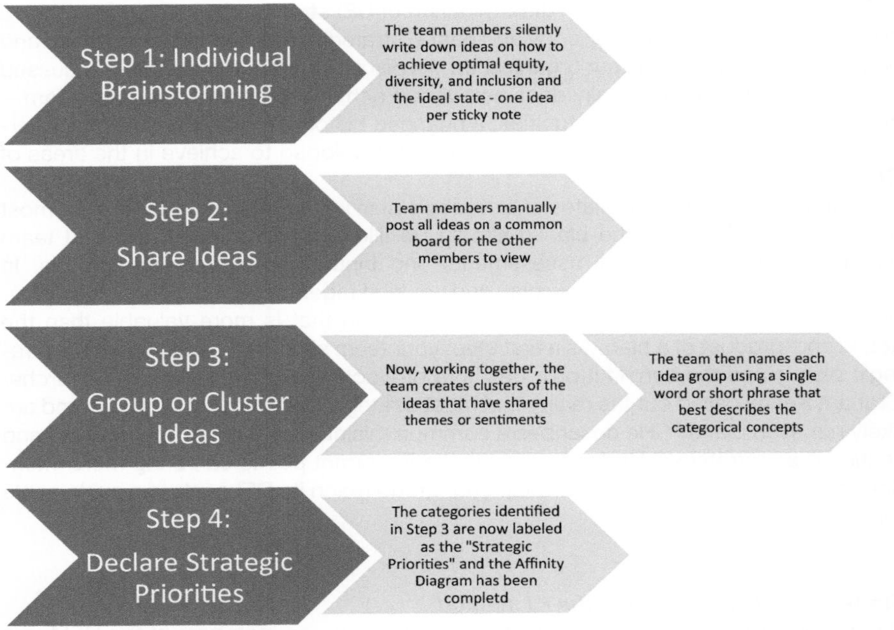

Fig. 1. Steps of the K-J technique to facilitate collective team brainstorming toward the identification of strategic diversity, equity, and inclusion priorities. This phase of the exercise is also referred to as the creation of an affinity diagram. (*Adapted from* Lucid. K-J Technique.2023, Retrieved from https://www.lucidmeetings.com/glossary/kj-technique.)

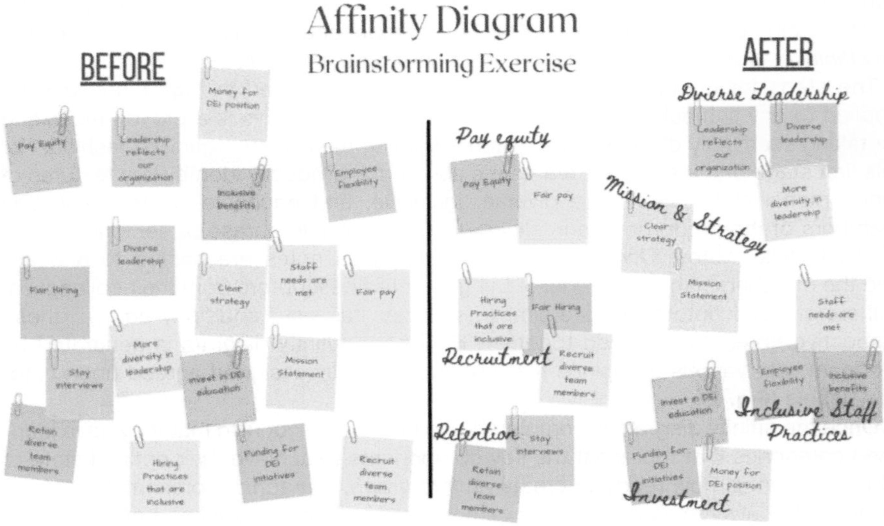

Fig. 2. Affinity diagram creation. Initially, the ideas generated from the brainstorm appear random and disorganized. The team works together to group similar ideas into clusters and then creates their own labels for the groupings, forming categories which will be declared as the strategic priorities.

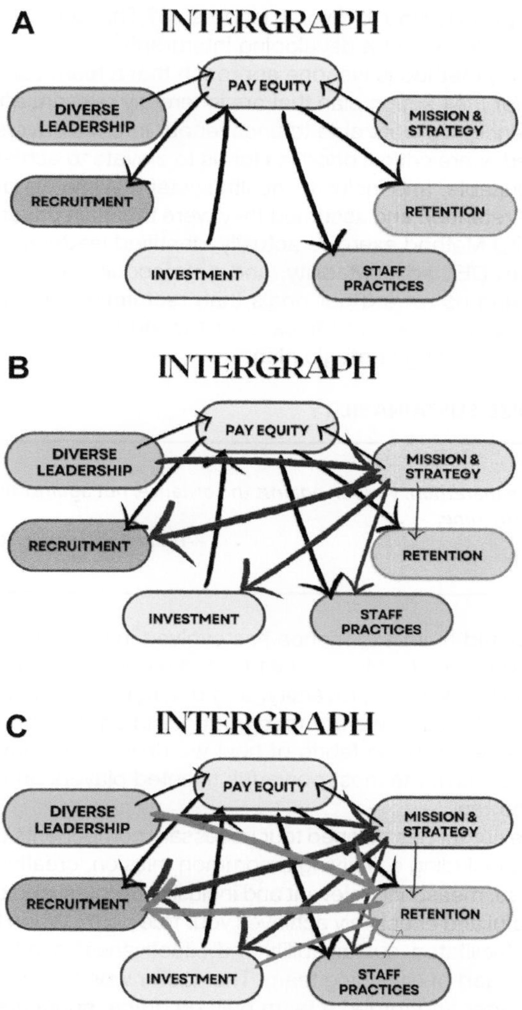

Fig. 3. Intergraph creation. Using the categories generated from the affinity diagram, a team can construct an intergraph to identify the key drivers toward attaining their diversity, equity, and inclusion (DEI) goals. Each individual category is compared to the rest, with the team considering in which direction the relationship arrow should be drawn. In (*A*), the black arrows compare "Pay Equity" to the remaining categories and identify the "driver" and the "receiver" of the pair through the direction of the arrows. In (*B*), the purple arrows compare "Mission and Strategy" to the remaining categories. In (*C*), the red arrows show the relationship between "Recruitment" and the other categories. This continues until each relationship direction between all the categories is determined. At the end of the exercise, the categories with the most arrows departing from them are considered the top drivers, and the categories with the most arrows pointing toward them are considered the top receivers.

equity? Or does pay equity lead to diverse leadership? This decision will be unique for each environment. A graphic of a developing intergraph is shown in **Fig. 3**(A–C).

In summary, the KJ Method is just one approach that a team can take to co-create strategic priorities for their action plan that are inherently relevant and insightful. From our group's experience, we were able to uncover our internal drivers that, while traditionally underscored, were critical priorities for us to elevate to achieve our mission toward a diverse, equitable, and inclusive health system. While we previously focused on recruitment and retention and assumed they were the main drivers toward diversity and inclusion, the KJ Method exercise actually identified leadership training, pay equity, investment into DEI, accountability, and data acquisition as areas much more instrumental in driving us toward our goals than recruitment. Most importantly, this discovery was created by us and for us, and therefore garnered broad buy-in for the execution of the resulting strategic plan.

SUMMARY: OPTIMIZE SUSTAINABILITY

> *When you run the marathon, you run against the distance, not against the other runners and not against the time.*
>
> *—Haile Gebrselassie (Olympic runner)*

The DEI leadership and team experience has evolved in response to a very dynamic state of change in our society. More industries are recognizing the power of incorporating lenses of equity, inclusion, diversity, and belonging into their operational business domains. In health care, we are recognizing and embracing the importance of integrating these lenses into the fabric of how we deliver care and build our teams. As in sports, you can have the most powerful, talented players on a team, but endurance is just as important.

In this review, the author has outlined four necessary components of empowering DEI leaders and teams, including solidifying a common mission, creating value around the team and its purpose, measuring relevant and inclusive outputs, and co-creating a strategy that is meaningful and effectively achieves your true north. When these components are combined and facilitated, sustainability and effectiveness can be increased.

We all want to be part of a winning team. The author would suggest that if you have supported a DEI leader and forged a team built on grace, connectedness, and intentional humanism, you have already won.

Onward.

ACKNOWLEDGEMENT

I would like to acknowledge my father, the late, great Charley Taylor - a former NFL Professional football player, NFL Hall of Famer, and an inspiration for many. As one of the first Black players to integrate the Washington Football Team in the 1960s, soon after Bobby Mitchell, his superhuman talents, leadership, and grace paved the way for others. Breaking these barriers, and many records, took the team to new heights that are still recognizable today. His legacy will continue to inspire all of us.

DISCLOSURE

Consultant, Johnson & Johnson DePuy Synthes. Other relationships/Speaker: Stryker, Total Joint Orthoapedics, Exactech.

REFERENCES

1. Cutter C, Weber L. Demand for chief diversity officers is high. so is turnover. Wall St J 2020.
2. Taylor E, Dacus R, Oni J, et al. An introduction to the orthopaedic diversity leadership consortium. J Bone Joint Surg 2022;104(72):1–4.
3. Ely R, Thomas D. Getting serious about diversity: enough already with the business case. Brighton, MA: Harvard Business Review; 2020.
4. (WHO), W. H. (2010). Framework for Action on Interprofessional Education & Collaborative Practice. Geneva.
5. McLaney E, Morassaei S, Hughes L, et al. A framework for interprofessional team collaboration in a hospital setting: Advancing team competencies and behaviours. Healthc Manage Forum 2022;35(2):112–7.
6. Braveman, P. A. (2017, May 17). What is health equity? and what difference does a definition make? Retrieved from Robert Wood Johnson Foundation: https://www.rwjf.org/en/library/research/2017/05/what-is-health-equity-.html.
7. Page S. The diversity bonus: how great teams pay off in the knowledge economy. Princeton, NJ: Princeton University Press; 2017.
8. McKinsey. (2020). Diversity Wins: How Inclusion Matters.
9. Gomez L, Bernet P. Diversity improves performance and outcomes. J Natl Med Assoc 2019;111(4):383–92.
10. Laurencin C, Murray M. An american crisis: the lack of black men in medicine. J Racial Ethn Health Disparities 2017;4(3):317–21.
11. NFL-Flag. How to create a winning flag football playbook 2023. Available at: https://nflflag.com/coaches/default/flag-football-rules/football-playbook.
12. Kenny G. Your strategic plans probably aren't strategic, or even plans. Harvard Business Review; 2018. Available at: https://hbr.org/2018/04/your-strategic-plans-probably-arent-strategic-or-even-plans.
13. Scupin R. The KJ method: A technique for analyzing data derived from Japanese ethnology. J Hum Rights 1997;56(2):233–7.

Printed and bound by CPI Group (UK) Ltd, Croydon, CR0 4YY
08/05/2025
01864749-0007